医学影像技术专业英语阅读与论文写作

（中英文对照）

王骏　周桂　徐娟　主编

东南大学出版社
SOUTHEAST UNIVERSITY PRESS
·南京·

内容提要

编者针对医学影像技术在校学生与在职人员提高英文阅读与写作水平的需要，围绕 CR、DR、CT、磁共振、PACS、辐射防护等医学影像技术学的相关理论与前沿知识，分题名、摘要、关键词、引言、正文、结论、致谢 7 部分，对医学影像技术英文论文的阅读和写作要点、技巧进行详细讲解。在编写结构上，学习、自测、自测答案相结合，内容设置循序渐进。如果按照作者设置，每天学一点，每天进步一点，坚持 5 个月，专业英语阅读与写作水平肯定会有很大提升。本书适合影像技术系学生、影像技术工作者学习使用。

图书在版编目(CIP)数据

医学影像技术专业英语阅读与论文写作 / 王骏，周桔，徐娟主编．—南京：东南大学出版社，2016. 12（2021.8 重印）

ISBN 978-7-5641-6680-9

Ⅰ．①医… Ⅱ．①王… ②周… ③徐… Ⅲ．①影像诊断－英语－阅读教学 ②影像诊断－英语－论文－写作

Ⅳ．① R445

中国版本图书馆 CIP 数据核字（2016）第 197464 号

医学影像技术专业英语阅读与论文写作

出版发行 东南大学出版社
出 版 人 江建中
社　　址 南京市四版楼 2 号（邮编 210096）
印　　刷 兴化印刷有限责任公司
经　　销 全国各地新华书店
开　　本 787 mm × 1092 mm 1/16
印　　张 12
字　　数 308 千字
版　　次 2016 年 12 月第 1 版 2021 年 8 月第 2 次印刷
书　　号 ISBN 978-7-5641-6680-9
定　　价 39.00 元

编者名单

主　编

王　骏　南京军区南京总医院（南京大学附属金陵医院）
周　桔　江苏广播电视大学
徐　娟　南京大学

副主编

陈　峰　海南省人民医院
李媛媛　中国药科大学
吴虹桥　南京医科大学常州市妇幼保健院
张文杰　解放军第 81 医院
刘小艳　南通大学附属医院

编　委（排名不分先后）

王　骏　南京军区南京总医院（南京大学附属金陵医院）
陈　峰　海南省人民医院
汤万鑫　四川卫生康复职业学院
岳文军　川北医学院附属医院
郭晋纲　山西医科大学附属肿瘤医院
刘小艳　南通大学附属医院
徐　娟　南京大学
李媛媛　中国药科大学
周　桔　江苏广播电视大学
吴虹桥　南京医科大学常州市妇幼保健院
张文杰　解放军第 81 医院

参编者（排名不分先后）

吴　寒　石瑞峰　张思裕　张　弛　崔丹婷　吴龙云　李　勰
吴文秀　朱雁铃　计忠伟　王　子　陆苑婷　戴亚婕　龙　柳
黄惠君　冯　倩　梁俊媚　林园凯　马　斯　陈凯填　胡振斌
黄杰茂　吴佳偿　李欣颖　杨凌乔　莫新海

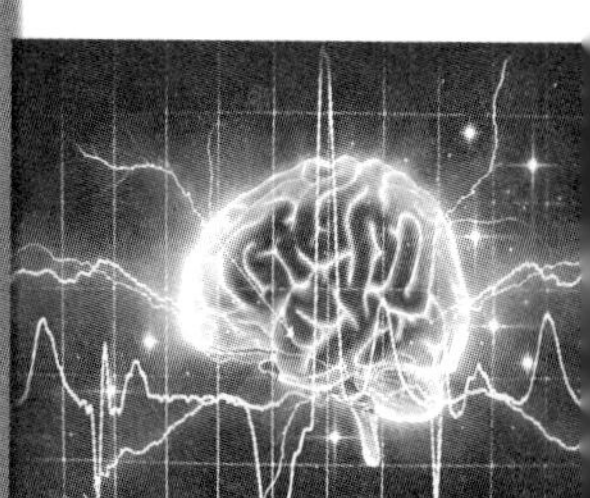

前 言

英语，是现代人工作、学习、生活、交流所必须掌握的一门应用语言，便于人们之间的沟通与了解、增进友谊、拉近距离，尤其是在当今的互联网 +、移动通信及云技术应用中则更是如此。

作为医学的一门分支学科，医学影像技术学的主要仪器、设备来自海外，其包含的知识涉及面广，不仅包括电子、电工、暗室化学和计算机与信息学知识，还包含生理、病理、解剖、成像技术与影像诊断知识等。这给我们在阅读参考文献或仪器说明书时带来巨大困难，常常需要借助公用辞典、科技辞典、医学辞典。作为一名放射师，如果没有较强的英文能力，其发展空间往往受限。

记得我在 20 世纪 90 年代初期，为了能了解国际上医学影像技术学发展动态，常到医院图书馆翻阅国际上著名的原版医学影像学期刊 *Radiology*（《放射学杂志》）、*AJR*（《美国放射学杂志》）、*BJR*（《英国放射学杂志》）、*EJR*（《欧洲放射学杂志》）等十余种，基本上是每期必览，并把一些重点文章复印后带回家慢慢咀嚼、消化、吸收，以不断强化自己的医疗、教学、科研能力。

刚开始接触专业英语文献时，常常是费了老鼻子劲儿才翻译了一小段，还驴唇不对马嘴，尤其是面对我们还没有的仪器、设备，翻译无异于“炼狱”。真想放弃！但身边的一位同事讲道：“如果你现在不进入专业英语，这辈子也就不用再想了！”外面的世界很精彩，不想落伍的我开始了艰难跋　涉：针对一个个词汇、一句句话、一段段文字，发扬“蚂蚁啃骨头”的精神。

最初，我从翻译短篇开始，我的老前辈们是踏踏实实做

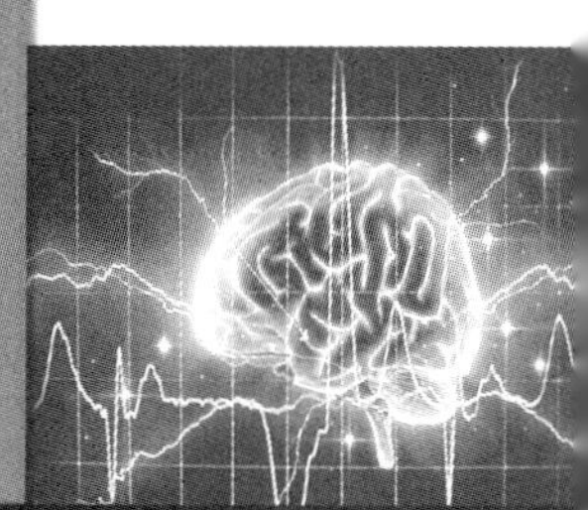

学问的人，不收任何报酬地就像对待小学生作文一样帮我逐字逐句地修改，往往一篇译文改下来已面目全非。通过翻译，我了解到国外科研的一些最新动态，学习了不少医学影像技术学的新理论、新知识、新装备、新技术以及诸多的科研方法，从中体会到作者严谨的科研态度，当然也提高了我的专业英文水平，使我科研论文的数量、质量都在不断地提高。

有时前辈们也会碰到个别翻译不准确的词语，他们一点也不敷衍，明确告诉我这里翻得不太好，可以到图书馆再查一查，再问问其他专家。于是我就找图书管理员，打开书柜，找最厚的英文辞海。慢慢地，我在国内著名的《国外医学临床放射学分册》《国外医学放射医学核医学分册》《国外医学医院管理分册》期刊上发表摘要、综述等，甚至在同一期期刊上刊登我翻译的三篇译稿。1992年、1993年我的科研论文入选亚洲放射技师大会、亚太放射技师大会、国际放射技师大会等，时至今日已发展到有多部译著，甚至专业英语翻译已成为我学习、工作、生活中的一部分。

随着时代的发展与要求，作为14亿的人口大国，要想站在国际舞台上亮相、出“声”显“影”，展示我国的学术水平与才华，这就更离不开专业英语的学习与提高。为此，该书从如何写论文的角度出发，全英汉对照学习专业英语，并对常见格式进行了归纳、总结。内容涵盖CR、DR、多排探测器CT、磁共振成像、DSA、PACS、QA、QC、安全防护等。从现在开始每天学习，每天进步一点点，哪怕就是进步1%，5个月下来定会受益匪浅。

当然，因时间和我们的学术水平有限，书中定有不少错误，还望广大同仁与学生通过微信（1145486363、骏哥哥）、E-mail（yingsong@sina.com）、医学影像健康网（www.mih365.com）、微信公众平台（mih365、医学影像健康网）发来您的批评与指正，以鞭策我们做得更好。最后，借此机会，感谢所有参编人员的无私奉献！

谨以此书献给正在医学影像技术学路上奋斗的人们！

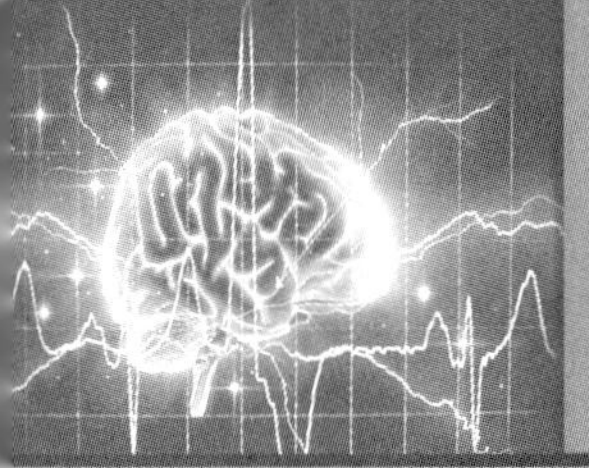

全军医学影像中心

南京军区南京总医院

南京大学附属金陵医院

王骏

2016年5月

目录

第 1 章 题名（Title）

第 2 章 摘要（Abstract）

第 3 章 关键词（Key words）

第 4 章 引言（Introduction）

第 5 章 正文（Body）

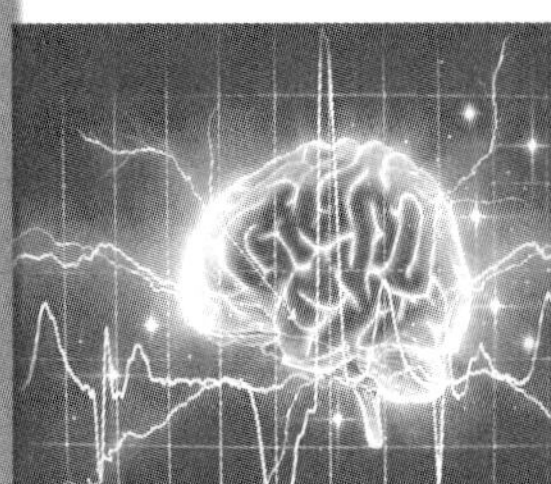

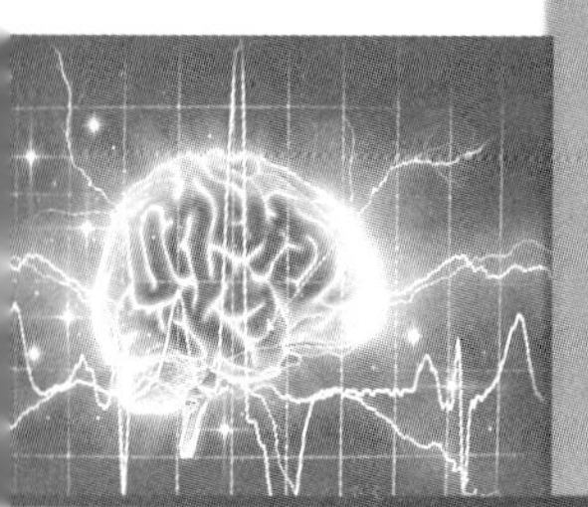

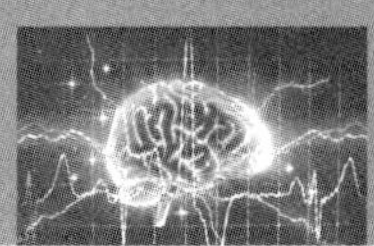

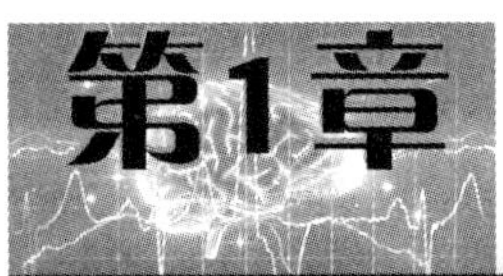

第1章　题名（Title）

题名是一篇文章的灵魂，一篇科研论文的展开均是围绕题名进行的。因此，题名要突出显示文章所要研究的内涵，要使读者透过题名能够判断作者所研究的内容。所以，作者不仅要通过题名来告知读者该篇文章的研究核心，而且还要通过题名抓住读者的眼球，吸引读者的注意，这就要求题名言简意赅，起到引导的作用。由此可见，题名要准确、简洁、全面地反映作者研究的主题思想，专一而有信息性。

一般来讲，英文题名不超过 120 个英文字符（包括空格），要有助于选定关键词，提供检索方便、实用的信息，如研究对象、研究方法、研究结果等。英文题名的书写格式有两种：第一种，每个词的第一个字母大写，虚词小写；第二种，仅题名第一个字母大写，其余小写。当然，专有名词、通用的缩略语也要大写。在题名上出现的缩略语，一定是约定俗成、人人皆知的，如计算机断层扫描用 “CT” 表示，磁共振用 “MR” 表示，图像存储与通讯系统用 “PACS” 表示，这样不仅能精简句式，还相当醒目。此外，还要注意名词的单、复数及可数与不可数。

一、　简洁句

科研文章无论是述评、综述，还是论著，其题名都要简明扼要。题名大多由名词性短语构成，也有少数题名是完整的句子，在这里统称为简洁句。通常，简洁句采用一些介词来指明题名内各名词及名词性词组间的逻辑关系，如 in, at, on, for, of, with, to; 也可以运用动词，如 use; 甚至，还可以采用 “-” 构成词组，如 -based。

第 1 天

学习

1. Chest Radiography

胸部 X 线摄影

chest [tʃest] *n.* 胸、胸廓　　　radiography [ˌredi'ɔgrəfi] *n.* X 线摄影

2. Memory Artifact Related to Selenium-based Digital Radiography System
   基于硒的数字 X 线摄影系统的记忆伪影
   artifact ['ɑ:tifækt]=artefact *n.* 伪影　　selenium [si'li:niəm] *n.* 硒
   Digital Radiography 数字 X 线摄影，简称 DR　　system ['sistim 'sistəm] *n.* 系统
3. Compression Device to Reduce Motion Artifacts at Contrast-enhanced MR Imaging in the Breast
   乳腺对比增强 MR 成像中采用压迫装置以减少移动伪影
   compression [kəm'preʃən] *n.* 压缩、加压、压力
   device [di'vais] *n.* 装置、设备、器件
   motion ['məuʃn] *n.* 运动、移位　　contrast-enhanced 对比增强
   MR Imaging 磁共振成像　　breast [brest] *n.* 乳房、乳腺

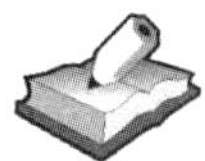
自测

1. 计算机 X 线摄影中的伪影
2. 裂隙扫描直接数字乳腺 X 线摄影的移动伪影

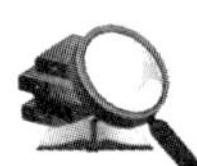
答案

1. Artifacts Found in Computed Radiography
   Computed Radiography 计算机 X 线摄影，简称 CR
2. Motion Artifact Seen on Slot-Scanning Direct Digital Mammography
   slot-scanning 裂隙扫描　　mammography [mæ'mɔgrəfi] *n.* 乳腺 X 线摄影

第 2 天

学习

1. Reference Lines for Oblique Axial MR Imaging of the Brain
   参考线在颅脑斜轴位 MR 成像中的应用
   reference lines 参考线　　oblique [ə'bli:k] *a.* 斜的，倾斜的
   axial ['æksiəl] *a.* 轴的，轴向的　　brain [brein] *n.* 脑
2. A CT-Compatible and MR-Compatible Reference Marker Box for Use with Stereotaxic Frames
   CT、MR 相容性参考标记箱在立体定向中的应用
   compatible [kəm'pætəbl] *a.* 相容的　　marker ['mɑ:kə] *n.* 标记
   stereotaxic [ˌstiəriəu'tæksik] *a.* 立体定位的　　frame [freim] *n.* 框架
3. MR-guided Biopsy of Suspect Breast Lesions with a Simple Stereotaxic Add-on Device

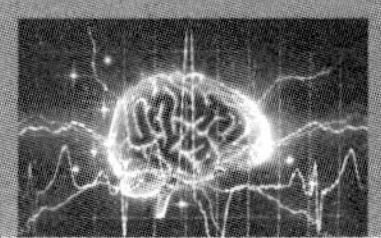

for Surface Coils
用 MR 表面线圈外加简单立体定向装置引导可疑乳腺病变穿刺活检
guide [gaid] *vt.* 引导　　suspect [səs'pekt] *vt.* 怀疑
biopsy ['baiɔpsi] *n.*,*vt.* 活检：aspiration biopsy，needle biopsy 针吸活检；take a biopsy 做活检
lesion ['li:ʒn] *n.* 损害、损伤　　surface coil 表面线圈

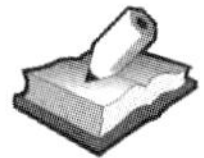 自测

1. 采用弛豫增强快速采集行腰椎 MR 脊髓造影
2. 利用固定装置工作间进行乳腺 X 线照相普查
3. 乳腺 X 线照片普查的影像质量对临床结果的影响

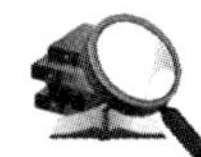 答案

1. Rapid Lumbar Spine MR Myelography Using Rapid Acquisition with Relaxation Enhancement
   lumbar ['lʌmbə] *a.* 腰的　　spine [spain] *n.* 脊柱
   myelography [ˌmaiə'lɔgrəfi] *n.* 脊髓造影术　　acquisition [ˌækwi'ziʃən] *n.* 获取、采集
   relaxation [ˌri:læk'seiʃən] *n.* 弛豫
2. Screening Mammography in Fixed Facility Workplace
   fixed [fikst] *a.* 固定的　　workplace *n.* 工作场所
   facility [fə'siliti] *n.* 容易、方便、灵活、装置（常为复数）
   screening ['skri:niŋ] *n.* 筛选、审查；screen ['skri:n] *n.* 屏；fluorescent screen 荧光屏、荧光板，intensifying screen 增感屏
3. Effect of Image Quality of Screening Mammography on Clinical Outcome
   image quality 影像质量
   effect [i'fekt] *n.* 作用、效应、影响；to have no effect，without effect 无效；with effect 有效；to the best effect 最有效地
   clinical ['klinikəl] *a.* 临床的、临床上的　　outcome ['autkʌm] *n.* 结果

第 3 天

 学习

1. File Management in a Radiology Department
   放射科的档案管理
   file [fail] *n.* 文件、档案　　Radiology Department 放射科

2. Teleradiology Using Consumer-Oriented Low-Cost Computer Hardware and Software
   远程放射学采用面向消费者的低成本计算机硬、软件
   teleradiology 远程放射学　　low-cost 低成本的
   consumer-oriented 面向消费者的　　computer hardware and software 计算机硬软件
3. A Simple Method of Capturing PACS and Other Radiographic Images for Digital Teaching Files or Other Image Repositories
   为数字教学文件或其他影像储存提取 PACS 及其他 X 线照片影像的一种简易方法
   method ['meθəd] *n.* 方法　　capture ['kæptʃə] *n./vt.* 捕捉、收集
   Picture Archiving and Communication System 图像存储与通讯系统，简称 PACS
   radiographic [ˌreidiəu'græfik] *a.* 放射摄影的、X 线摄影的
   repository [ri'pɔzətri] *n.* 仓库、资源丰富地区

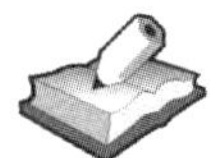
自测

影像存储与通讯系统与病人检查记录的丢失

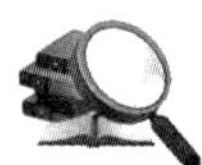
答案

Picture Archiving and Communication System (PACS) and the Loss of Patient's Examination Records

loss [lɔs　lɔ:s] *n.* 丢失、损失; loss of 损失　　patient ['peiʃənt] *n.* 病人、患者

第 4 天

学习

1. Actual Cost in Diagnostic Radiology
   放射诊断的实际成本
   diagnostic [ˌdaiəg'nɔstik] *a.* 诊断的
2. Radiation Cost of Helical High-Resolution Chest CT
   螺旋高分辨力胸部 CT 的辐射成本
   radiation [ˌreidi'eiʃən] *n.* 辐射、照射　　helical ['helikl] *a.* 螺旋的
   high-resolution 高分辨率　computed tomography 计算机断层扫描，简称 CT
3. Radiation Risk is Linear with Dose at Low Doses
   在低剂量下辐射风险与剂量成线性关系
   dose [dəus] *n.* 剂量　　linear ['liniə] *a.* 线型的，线的

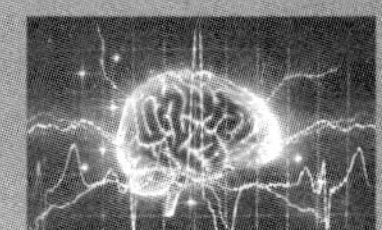

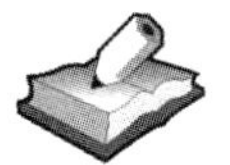
自测

1. 低剂量放射风险
2. CT 检查的技术成本
3. 适当剂量率的电离辐射使人更长寿

答案

1. The Risk of Low Dose Radiation
2. Technical Cost of CT Scan
3. Moderate Dose Rate Ionizing Radiation Increases Longevity
   moderate ['mɔdərət] *a.* 适度的、有节制的　　　ionizing radiation 电离辐射
   longevity [lɔn'dʒevəti] *n.* 长寿

为了使标题一目了然，常会在题目中采用缩略词，但此缩略词一定要是行业内认可的最常见词汇，如 CR（计算机 X 线摄影）、DR（数字 X 线摄影）、CT（计算机断层扫描）、MDCT（多排探测器 CT）、MRI（磁共振成像）、DSA（数字减影血管造影）等。

第 5 天

学习

1. General Principles of MDCT
   多排探测器 CT 的一般原理
2. PET in the Follow-up of Differentiated Thyroid Cancer
   PET 随访鉴别甲状腺癌
   differentiate [difə'renʃieit] *vt.* 鉴别
   thyroid ['θairɔid] *a.* 甲状腺
3. Cumulative Radiation Exposure and Cancer Risk Estimates in Emergency Department Patients Undergoing Repeat or Multiple CT
   在急诊科患者进行重复或多次 CT 检查累积射线曝光与癌症风险评估
   Emergency Department 急诊科

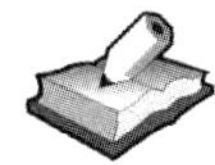
自测

1. 儿科胸部 CT 降低放射剂量策略的评价
2. 回顾性心电门控冠状动脉 CT 血管造影在低放射曝光协议中的图像质量

3. 全视野数字乳腺X线放大摄影（2倍）与数字乳腺放大显示（1.8倍）对微小钙化的诊断

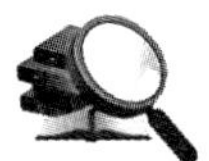 答案

1. Evaluation of a Radiation Dose Reduction Strategy for Pediatric Chest CT
   pediatric [ˌpi:di'ætrik] *a.* 儿科学的
2. Image Quality in a Low Radiation Exposure Protocol for Retrospectively ECG-Gated Coronary CT Angiography
3. Zooming Method(× 2.0) of Digital Mammography vs Digital Magnification View(× 1.8) in Full-field Digital Mammography for the Diagnosis of Microcalcifications

二、 副题名

在题名不能完全表达作者意图时，或是为了突出作者所研究的领域、范围、方法、结果与别人不同时，通常采用副题名来陈述。副题名可用来突出病例数目、研究重点、研究方法，对主题名做进一步的说明、补充，并用冒号或破折号与主题名隔开。

第6天

 学习

1. Digital Chest Radiography：Effect of Temporal Subtraction on Detection Accuracy
   数字胸部X线摄影：时间减影在检测准确性中的作用
   temporal subtraction 时间减影
2. Flat-Panel Display (LCD) versus High-Resolution Gray-Scale Display (CRT) for Chest Radiography：An Observer Preference Study
   胸部X线摄影在平面显示器(LCD)与高分辨力灰阶显示器(CRT)的主观对照研究
   flat-panel display 平面显示器　　gray-scale 灰阶
3. Routine Chest Radiography Using a Flat-Panel Detector：Image Quality at Standard Detector Dose and 33% Dose Reduction
   采用平板探测器的常规胸部X线摄影：标准探测器剂量和降低33%剂量的影像质量
   routine chest radiography 常规胸部X线摄影　　flat-panel detector 平板探测器

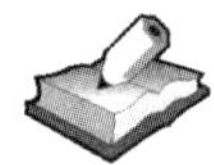 自测

1. 胸部数字X线摄影与传统X线摄影的对比：利用临床CT对照研究大面积硅平板探测器的诊断性能

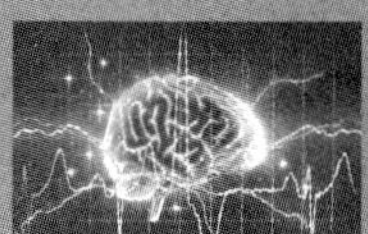

2. 大面积非晶体硅平板探测器的临床对比研究：胸部 X 线摄影的影像质量和解剖结构的显示
3. 手和足的硒数字 X 线摄影与传统屏 - 片 X 线摄影的比较：主观比较

答案

1. Digital Radiography versus Conventional Radiography in Chest Imaging: Diagnostic Performance of a Large-Area Silicon Flat-Panel Detector in a Clinical CT Control Study
   conventional radiography 传统 X 线摄影
   silicon ['silikən] *n.* 硅
   control [kən'trəul](controlled) *v.* 控制、管理；control study 对照研究
2. Clinical Comparative Study with a Large-Area Amorphous Silicon Flat-Panel Detector: Image Quality of Chest Radiography and Visibility of Anatomic Structures
   comparative [kəm'pærətiv] *a.* 比较的　　　amorphous silicon 非晶硅
   anatomic structures 解剖结构
3. Selenium-Based Digital Radiography versus Conventional Film-Screen Radiography of the Hands and Feet: A Subjective Comparison
   conventional film-screen radiography 传统屏 - 片 X 线摄影
   subjective [sʌb'dʒektiv] *a.* 主观的

第 7 天

学习

1. Direct Coronal CT of the Wrist: Helical Acquisition with Simplified Patient Positioning
   腕部直接冠状 CT：患者简单定位的螺旋扫描
   coronal ['kɔrənl] *a.* 冠状的　　　wrist [rist] *n.* 腕
   position [pə'ziʃən] *vt.* 给……定位
2. Image Quality and Dose Comparison among Screen-Film Computed Radiography, and CT Scanned Projection Radiography: Applications to CT Urography
   比较屏 - 片计算机 X 线摄影、CT 扫描照片的影像质量和剂量：在 CT 尿路造影术中的应用
   projection [prə'dʒekʃən] *n.* 投射、投影
   urography [juə'rɔgrəfi] *n.* 尿路造影术；intravenous urography 静脉尿路造影术，retrograde urography 逆行性尿路造影术
3. Dual-Source CT: Effect of Heart Rate, Heart Rate Variability, and Calcification on Image

Quality and Diagnostic Accuracy
双源 CT：心率、心率变化和钙化对图像质量和诊断精度的影响
dual-source CT 双源 CT　　calcification [ˌkælsifiˈkeiʃən] *n.* 钙化

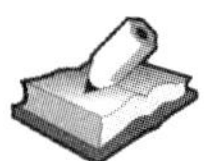 自测

1. 腹部螺旋 CT：每周扫描时间为 0.75 s 和 1 s 时的影像质量比较
2. 多排探测器 CT 冠状动脉血管造影：重建技术和心率对图像质量的影响
3. 使用双源 CT 双能量技术的 Xe 通气 CT：初步研究

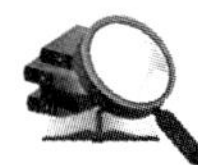 答案

1. Helical CT of the Abdomen：Comparison of Image Quality between Scan Times of 0.75 and 1 Sec per Revolution
abdomen [ˈæbdəmen　æbˈdəumen] *n.* 腹部；acute abdomen 急腹症
revolution [ˌrevəˈlu:ʃn] *n.* 循环、周期
2. Multi–Detector Row CT Coronary Angiography：Influence of Reconstruction Technique and Heart Rate on Image Quality
multi–detector row CT 多排探测器 CT　　coronary angiography 冠状动脉血管造影
reconstruction [ˌri:kənˈstrʌkʃn] *n.* 重建
3. Xenon Ventilation CT with a Dual-Energy Technique of Dual-Source CT：Initial Experience
xenon [ˈzenɔn] *n.* 氙　　ventilation [ˌventiˈleiʃən] *n.* 通气
dual-energy technique 双能量技术

第 8 天

1. Urinary Calculi on Computed Radiography：Comparison of Observer Performance with Hard-Copy versus Soft-Copy Images on Different Viewer Systems
计算机 X 线摄影中的泌尿道结石：在硬拷贝与软拷贝不同观察系统上比较观察者的喜好
urinary [ˈjuərinəri] *a.* 尿的
calculus [ˈkælkjuləs](复数 calculuses 或 calculi) *n.* 结石
hard-copy 硬拷贝
soft-copy 软拷贝

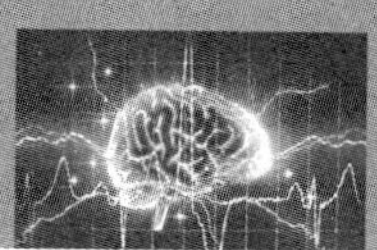

2. Detection of Small Low-Contrast Objects in Mammography: Effect of Viewbox Masking and Luminance
   在乳腺 X 线摄影中小的低对比病灶的诊断：观片灯遮蔽和亮度的作用
   luminance ['lu:minəns] *n.* 亮度
3. ROC Curve Analysis of Lesion Detectability on Phantoms: Comparison of Digital Mammography with Conventional Mammography
   在体模上病灶诊断能力的 ROC 曲线分析：数字乳腺 X 线摄影与传统乳腺 X 线摄影的比较
   ROC curve analysis　ROC 曲线分析　　phantom ['fæntəm] *n.* 体模

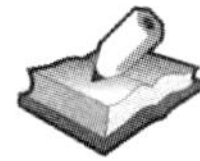

自测

乳腺 X 线摄影普查：临床影像质量和间隔期乳腺癌的风险

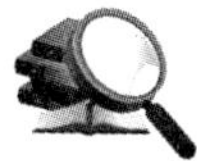

答案

Screening Mammography: Clinical Image Quality and the Risk of Interval Breast Cancer

interval ['intəvl] *n.* 间隔、间期

cancer ['kænsə] *n.* 癌、癌症、恶性肿瘤；cancer in situ 原位癌

第 9 天

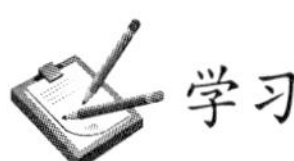

学习

1. Work Flow Redesign: The Key to Success When Using PACS
   重新设计工作流程：使用 PACS 成功的关键
   work flow 工作流程　　redesign [ˌri:di'zain] *v.* 重新设计
2. MRI of Meniscal Lesions: Soft-Copy (PACS) and Hard-Copy Evaluation versus Reviewer Experience
   半月板撕裂的磁共振成像：软拷贝（PACS）和硬拷贝评价与读片人经验相比较
   meniscal ['məniskl] *a.* 半月板的
3. Severe Acute Respiratory Syndrome: Avoiding the Spread of Infection in a Radiology
   严重急性呼吸综合征（SARS）：避免在放射科传播感染
   Severe Acute Respiratory Syndrome 严重急性呼吸综合征

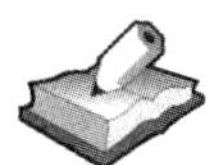

自测

在万维网上传输医学影像为临床急诊服务：1 例报告

答案

Transferring Medical Images on the World Wide Web for Clinical Emergency Management: a Case Report

transfer ['trænsfə:](transferred, transferring) *v.* 传输

medical ['medikəl] *a.* 医学的、医疗的、内科的　　the world wide web 万维网

emergency [i'mə:dʒənsi] *n.* 急症、紧急　　a case report　1 例报告

第 10 天

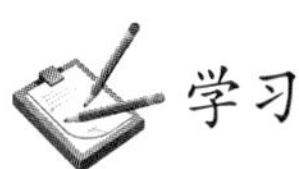

学习

1. CT Dose Index and Patient Dose:They Are Not the Same Thing
   CT 剂量指数与患者剂量：它们不是一回事儿
2. Whole-Body PET/CT Scanning:Estimation of Radiation Dose and Cancer Risk
   全身 PET/CT 扫描：放射剂量的评估与癌症风险

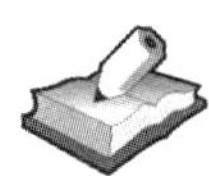

自测

1. 图像存储与通讯系统：放射学信息技术
2. 泌尿系结石：降低 50% 和 75% 的 CT 放射剂量——灵敏度的影响

答案

1. Picture Archiving and Communication Systems:Information Technology in Radiology
2. Urinary Calculi:Radiation Dose Reduction of 50% and 75% at CT—Effect on Sensitivity

第 11 天

学习

1. Prospective Gating with 320-MDCT Angiography:Effect of Volume Scan Length on Radiation Dose
   前瞻性门控 320 排探测器 CT 血管造影：容积扫描长度对放射剂量的影响
2. Receiver Operating Characteristic(ROC) Analysis:Basic Principles and Applications in Radiology

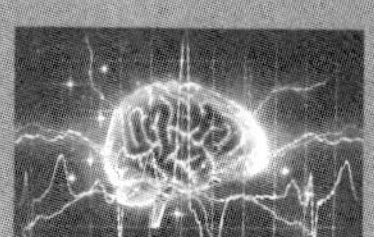

受试者作业特征曲线（ROC）分析：基本原理及其在放射学的应用

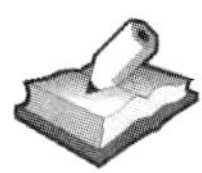 自测

1. CT 结肠造影筛查辐射相关癌症风险：风险与利益分析
2. 320 层 CT 神经成像：初步临床经验和影像质量评价

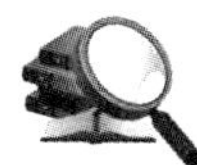 答案

1. Radiation-Related Cancer Risks from CT Colonography Screening:A Risk-Benefit Analysis
   colonography [ˌkəulə'nɔgrəfi] *n.* 结肠造影术
2. 320-Slice CT Neuroimaging:Initial Clinical Experience and Image Quality Evaluation

第 12 天

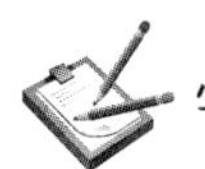 学习

1. Vascular Enhancement and Image Quality of MDCT Pulmonary Angiography in 400 Cases:Comparison of Standard and Low Kilovoltage Settings
   多排探测器 CT 肺血管造影的 400 例血管增强和影像质量：标准千伏与低千伏对比研究
   angiography [ˌændʒi'grəfi] *n.* 血管造影术
2. Evaluation of Image Quality and Radiation Dose in Adolescent Thoracic Imaging:64-Slice is Preferable to 16-Slice Multislice CT
   对青少年胸部成像中影像质量和放射剂量的评价：64 层比 16 层多层 CT 更优越
   adolescent [ˌædə'lesənt] *a.* 青少年的

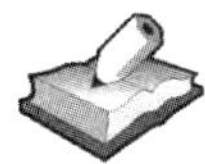 自测

1. 采用双回波 Dixon 技术的骨盆 T_1 加权脂肪抑制成像：初步临床经验
2. 全视野数字乳腺 X 线摄影计算机辅助检测：系列检查中的灵敏度与再显力

 答案

1. T_1-weighted Fat-suppressed Imaging of the Pelvis with a Dual-Echo Dixon Technique:Initial Clinical Experience
2. Computer-aided Detection in Full-Field Digital Mammography:Sensitivity and

Reproducibility in Serial Examinations

computer-aided detection 计算机辅助检测 (CAD)

第 13 天

用一个副题名不足以全面展示所表达的思想时，也可以采用第二个副题名延伸内涵，但这并不常见。

Renal Stone Assessment with Dual-Energy Multidetector CT and Advanced Postprocessing Techniques:Improved Characterization of Renal Stone Composition—Pilot Study

肾结石双能量多排探测器 CT 评价和先进后处理技术：提高肾结石成分的识别——潜展性研究

postprocessing 后处理

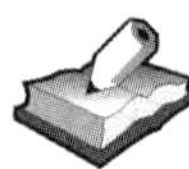

低管电压、高管电流多排探测器腹部 CT：采用适当的统计迭代重建算法改善图像质量和降低放射剂量——初步临床经验

Low-tube-voltage, High-tube-current Multidetector Abdominal CT：Improved Image Quality and Decreased Radiation Dose with Adaptive Statistical Iterative Reconstruction Algorithm—Initial Clinical Experience

iterative ['itərətiv] *a.* 迭代的

三、 疑问句

为了引起读者的关注，在述评中，往往会采用疑问句的形式来突出强调作者所阐述的主题思想，这样可引发读者的思考，而论著中一般不用。

第 14 天

1. CT and Computed Radiography：The Pictures Are Great, But Is the Radiation Dose

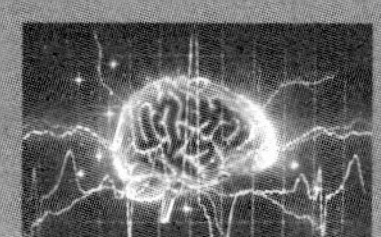

Greater Than the Required?

CT 与计算机 X 线摄影：图像质量好了，但放射剂量比所需的要大吗？

2. Cost, Value, and Price：What Is the Difference and Why Care?

成本、价值与价格：有什么差异？为什么关注？

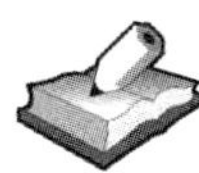 自测

CT 放射剂量：我们所面临的挑战？

 答案

Radiation Dose in CT：Are We Meeting the Challenge?

challenge ['tʃælindʒ] *n.* 挑战

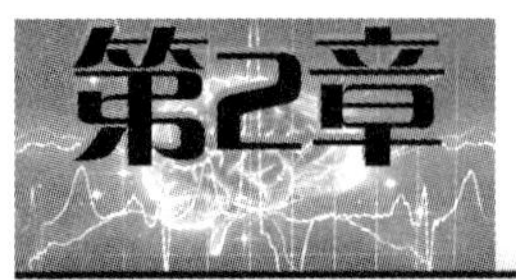

第2章 摘要（Abstract）

摘要是全文的重要组成部分，是对全文的高度浓缩。可以说，摘要就相当于一篇小文章，可以通过摘要让读者了解全文所研究的目的，通过什么方法进行科学研究，得出什么结果，结论怎样。相当于内容梗概，以利于读者检索。当然，摘要离不开概括性语言，但必须言之有物，切忌假、大、空，更不能加入主观见解、解释和评论性语言。通常摘要分为指示性摘要（indicative abstract）、报道性摘要（informative abstract）、报道-指示性摘要（informative-indicative abstract）、结构式摘要（structured abstract）。下面就结构式摘要进行详细阐述。

一、目　的

摘要中的目的与全文中的目的在写作方法上不是一回事，摘要中的目的往往就是一句话交待作者所须研究的意图是什么，或是为什么要开展这项研究。开门见山，直奔主题，不能大刀阔斧地畅谈学术背景与不足。通常有以下几种表达方法：

第 15 天

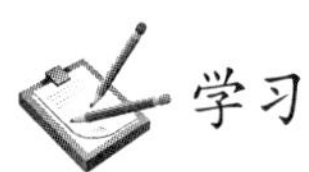

学习

第一种：采用“The objective of this study was to...”句式，或“The purpose of this study was to...”句式。

1. The objective of this study was to compare the diagnostic performance of a digital large-area silicon flat-panel detector with that of a conventional screen-film system in clinical chest imaging using abnormal findings documented by CT as the reference standard.
   该研究的目的是利用 CT 检查中异常发现作为参考标准比较数字大面积硅平板探测器与传统屏-片系统在临床胸部成像中的诊断性能。
   abnormal[æb'nɔ:ml]*a.* 异常的
2. The purpose of this study was to subjectively compare the visibility of normal anatomy

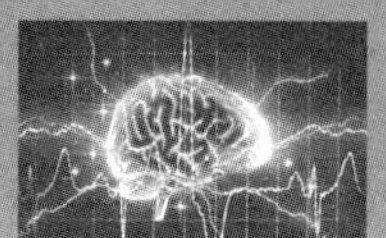

of the hands and feet using selenium-based digital radiography versus conventional film-screen (100-speed) radiography.

该研究的目的是采用以硒为基础的数字 X 线摄影相对于传统屏 - 片（速度为 100）X 线摄影主观比较手和足的正常解剖可见度。

the visibility of normal anatomy 正常解剖的可见度

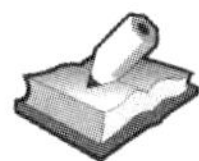

自测

1. The objective of this study was to compare clinical chest radiographs of a large-area, flat-panel digital radiography system with a conventional film-screen radiography system. The comparison was based on an observer preference study of image quality and visibility of anatomic structures.
2. The purpose of this study was to compare observer performance for detecting urinary calculi using abdominal computed radiography with hard-copy versus soft-copy images and with a high-resolution video monitor versus a liquid-crystal-display (LCD) monitor.

答案

1. 该研究的目的是比较大面积平板数字 X 线摄影系统与传统屏 - 片 X 线摄影系统的临床胸部 X 线照片。此比较基于影像质量与解剖结构可见度的观察者倾向的研究。
   flat-panel digital radiography system 平板数字 X 线摄影系统
   a conventional film-screen radiography system 传统屏 - 片 X 线摄影系统
   image quality 影像质量　　　visibility of anatomic structures 解剖结构的可见度
2. 该研究的目的是采用腹部计算机 X 线摄影比较硬拷贝与软拷贝影像以及高分辨率图像显示器与液晶显示器比较观察者诊断尿路结石的能力。
   a high-resolution video monitor 高分辨率图像显示器
   a liquid-crystal-display (LCD) monitor 液晶显示器

第 16 天

学习

第二种：采用 “To prospectively evaluate…” 句式，也可以直接用 “To evaluate…” 句式。

To prospectively evaluate the effect of heart rate, heart rate variability, and calcification on dual-source computed tomography (CT) image quality and to prospectively assess diagnostic accuracy of dual-source CT for coronary artery stenosis, by using invasive coronary angiography as the reference standard.

该研究利用双源 CT 影像质量评价心率、心率变化与钙化之间的关系，采用有创冠状动脉血管造影作为参考标准，评价双源 CT 对于冠状动脉狭窄诊断的精确性。

coronary artery stenosis 冠状动脉狭窄

invasive coronary angiography 有创冠状动脉血管造影

备注：在一句话中，同时出现两个“评价”时，在不影响语意的前提下尽可能换用一个词语表达，以活跃语言氛围而不显得死板。

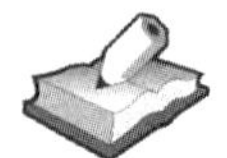
自测

To evaluate image quality and dose for abdominal imaging techniques that could be used as part of a computed tomographic (CT) urographic examination: screen-film (S-F) radiography or computed radiography (CR), performed with moving and stationary grids, and CT scanned projection radiography (CT SPR).

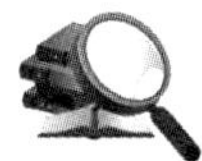
答案

评价使用 CT 尿路检查腹部成像技术，即使用移动或固定滤线栅进行屏 - 片（S-F）X 线摄影、计算机 X 线摄影（CR）、CT 扫描投影 X 线摄影（CT SPR）的影像质量与剂量之间的关系。

moving and stationary grids 移动或固定滤线栅

第 17 天

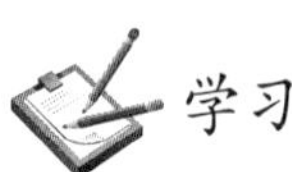
学习

第三种：采用“Our goal was to…”，或“Our objective was to…”格式。

Our goal was to determine the appearance of motion artifact when imaging an breast phantom using a digital slot- scanning system compared with a screen-film system.

我们的目的是采用与屏 - 片系统相比数字裂隙扫描系统乳腺体模成像移动伪影的显示。

motion artifact 移动伪影　　　　breast phantom 乳腺体模

a digital slot- scanning system 数字裂隙扫描系统

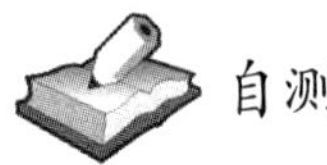
自测

Viewing conditions can affect an observer's performance in object detection. Our objective was to determine the effect of viewbox masking and luminance on the detection of small low-contrast objects revealed by mammography.

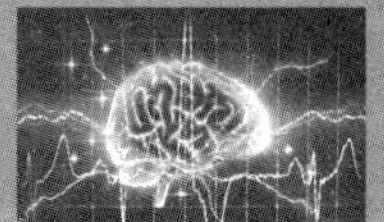

答案

观片条件能影响观察者在目标诊断方面的效果。我们的目的是确定观片灯遮蔽及其亮度在乳腺 X 线摄影中对低对比小的异常方面的诊断影响。

viewing conditions 观片条件

第 18 天

学习

其他一些句式，如："To improve…""To measure…"；也可以采用第一人称，如："We evaluated…"；甚至，还可以用主动语态介绍。

To improve early detection of disease in chest radiographs, the authors developed a digital processing technique that geometrically warps and subtracts a previous radiograph from a current radiograph to produce a temporal subtraction image. An observer test was performed to evaluate the effects of the temporal subtraction image technique on detection of interval change.

在胸部 X 线照片中，为改善疾病早期诊断，作者研发了几何卷积及从当前的 X 线照片减去以前的 X 线照片产生时间减影图像的数字处理技术。通过观察者测试来评价时间减影图像技术在诊断间隔性改变方面的作用。

chest radiographs 胸部 X 线照片

a digital processing technique 数字处理技术

temporal subtraction image 时间减影图像

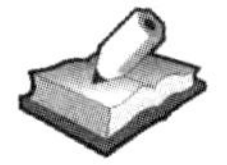

自测

To measure the technical cost of different categories of computed tomographic (CT) examinations.

答案

衡量不同类别的 CT 检查技术成本。

第 19 天

学习

The purpose of this article is to compare workflow efficiency between a conventional computed radiography(CR) system and a novel,portable,cassette-sized,and wireless flat-panel digital radiography(DR) system.

本文的目的是为了比较传统计算机 X 线摄影（CR）系统和新颖的、可移动的、暗盒式的、无线平板数字 X 线摄影（DR）系统之间的工作效率。

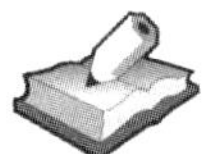 自测

我们研究的目的是，改变胸部 CT 扫描协议中使用低千伏策略，量化其对患者剂量、图像质量和图像噪声所产生的影响。

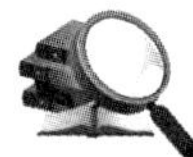 答案

The purpose of our study was to quantify the effect of changes made to the CT chest protocol on patient dose,image quality,and image noise when using a kilovoltage(kVp)-lowering strategy.

第 20 天

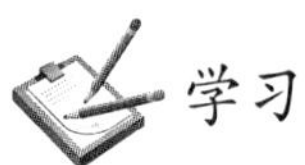 学习

There is a known risk from radiation.The objective of this article is to answer the following question regarding CT:Is there a risk of lowering the radiation exposure so low that the risk of missing a diagnosis from excessive noise in the image begins to exceed the risk of the radiation itself.

众所周知，辐射具有风险。这篇文章的目的是回答下列 CT 相关问题：放射曝光降得太低，所带来的图像噪声过度增加，致使漏诊的风险是否超过放射本身所带来的风险。

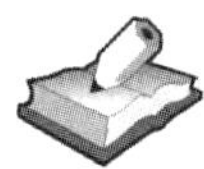 自测

采用 1.5T 磁共振（MR）系统，比较采用标准快速自旋回波 T_1 加权化学位移脂肪抑制获得的双回波 Dixon 技术水成像的图像质量，以评价骨盆疼痛患者。

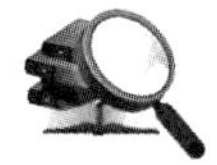 答案

To compare the image quality of water-only images generated from a dual-echo Dixon technique with that of standard fast spin-echo T_1-weighted chemical shift fat-suppressed images obtained in patients evaluated for pelvic pain with a 1.5-T magnetic resonance(MR) system.

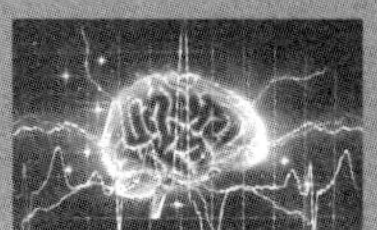

第 21 天

学习

1. 表达研究目的的常用句式如下：

The goal (aim) of this investigation was to... 该研究目的是……

This study was designed to... 该研究旨在……

This prospective study was performed to... 该前瞻性研究的目的是……

An attempt has been made to... 为了……而做试验

We (the authors) conducted a study to... 为了……我们进行了研究

To determine..., we studied... 为了确定……，我们研究了……

In an attempt to (in an effort to, in order to)..., we carried out a pilot study... 为了……，我们进行了……的初步研究

2. 表达研究目的的常用动词：evaluate（评价），examine（检查），determine（确定），explore（探索），test（测试），compare（比较），estimate（评估），assess（估价），investigate（调查）。

二、方　法

在方法中要阐明作者研究所采用的病例资料，如例数、年龄、性别等。研究方法的内容既要翔实，又不能完全展开，更不能空洞泛谈，要言之有物。

第 22 天

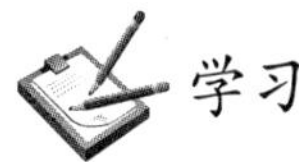

学习

Eighty patients (46 men and 34 women; age range, 18—91 years old; mean age, 63 years old) who underwent CT of the chest were examined with the new digital radiography system, which is based on a 43 cm × 43 cm silicon flat-panel detector, and with a conventional screen-film system, which is used routinely in clinical practice. Posteroanterior and lateral radiographs were obtained. Four radiologists analyzed the digital and conventional images separately for chest abnormalities and rated the images using a five-level scale of confidence; CT was used as the reference standard. Diagnostic value was assessed using receiver operating characteristic curves for each abnormality.

进行 CT 检查的 80 例患者（男 46 例、女 34 例，年龄范围：18 ~ 91 岁，平均年龄：63 岁）采用新的数字 X 线摄影系统（基于 43 cm × 43 cm 硅平板探测器）与传统屏 - 片系统进

行常规胸部检查。采用后前位与侧位 X 线照片。4 位放射学家分别就胸部异常用 5 个等级评分判断影像来分析数字与传统图像；采用 CT 作为参考标准。对各个异常利用受试者作业特性曲线评价诊断价值。

posteroanterior ['pɔstərəˌæn'tiəriə] *a.* 后前位的　　lateral ['lætərəl] *a.* 侧的

receiver operating characteristic curves 受试者作业特性曲线

注：第一个句子是复句，其中有三个定语从句，第一个从句 who underwent… 修饰 Eighty patients；第二个 which is based on… 修饰 new digital radiography system；第三个定语 which is used routinely in clinical practice 修饰 a conventional screen-film system。其中后面两个定语从句为对称结构，写长的句子时可以参考、借鉴。

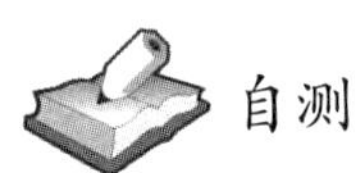

自测

The chest radiographs of 50 patients (age range, 16-79 years old; mean age, 57 years old) were obtained at two different detector dose levels. Digital images were taken from the same patients in posteroanterior and lateral views with detector doses of 2.5 μGy and 1.8 μGy, respectively, at 125 kVp tube voltage. The cesium iodide-amorphous silicon active-matrix imager had a panel size of 43 cm × 43 cm, a matrix of 3 000 × 3 000, and a pixel pitch of 143 μm. Images were presented in a random order to three independent radiologists who were unaware of the dose level at which the images had been obtained. They subjectively rated image quality on a 4-point scale. Statistical significance of differences was evaluated with Student's *t* test for paired samples (confidence level, 95%).

答案

利用两种不同探测器剂量获得 50 例（年龄范围：16 ~ 79 岁，平均年龄：57 岁）胸部 X 线照片。对于同一个患者进行后前位与侧位数字摄影，探测器剂量分别为 2.5 μGy 与 1.8 μGy，管电压为 125 kVp。碘化铯非晶硅激活矩阵平板尺寸为 43 cm × 43 cm，矩阵为 3 000 × 3 000，像素大小为 143 μm。3 位放射学家独自随机判断影像，但不知其剂量。他们依据 4 个级别判定影像质量。用配对 *t* 检验进行统计学分析（可信度为 95%）。

cesium iodide 碘化铯　　pitch [pitʃ] *n.* 螺距

matrix ['meitriks]（复数 matrices 或 matrixes）*n.* 基质、矩阵

a panel size 平板尺寸　　the dose level 剂量水平

Student's *t* test for paired samples 配对 *t* 检验　　confidence level 可信度

be unaware of 不知情　　tube voltage 管电压

第 23 天

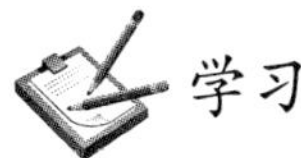
学习

1. 表达研究方法的常用句式如下。

   Using…(technique), we studied... 我们用……（技术）研究了……

   Using…, it was found that… 我们用……发现了……

   …was(were) measured using… 我们用……测定了……

   …was(were) analyzed by… 我们用……分析了……

   …measurements were made of… 测定了……

   …were randomly divided into…groups　……被随机分为……组

   …were separated into…groups, based on… 根据……,将……分为……组

   The groups were as follows… 分组如下……

2. 表达研究方法的常用动词：determine（测定）, investigate（研究）, demonstrate（证明）, examine（检查）, identify（鉴定）等。

三、结　果

结果就是作者对资料进行研究后所得出的数据,这里的数据是指对原始数据的高度概括,而不是单纯地将原始数据进行罗列,是得出结论的依据。

第 24 天

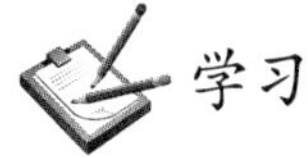
学习

In all categories, selenium-based digital images were rated equivalent to film-screen images by the five observers. Using the sum of the nine landmarks, four of the five observers rated the quality of selenium-based digital images superior to that of film-screen images.

对于所有类别, 5 位观察者判定以硒为基础的数字影像等同于屏 - 片影像。采用 9 个标记, 4 位观察者判定以硒为基础的数字影像质量优于屏 - 片影像质量。

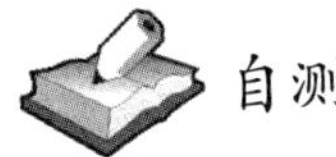
自测

No significant differences were found between the area under the receiver operating characteristic curve of the digital and that of the conventional radiography method for almost all investigated criteria. The only exception was mediastinal abnormalities, for which the digital method provided better results than the conventional method ($P < 0.05$).

答案

对照所有研究标准，数字 X 线摄影与传统 X 线摄影的受试者作业特性曲线下的面积无显著差异。只有纵隔病变数字方法比传统方法提供较好的结果 ($P < 0.05$)。

no significant differences 无显著差异　　mediastinal [ˌmi:diæs'tainl] *a*. 纵隔的

第 25 天

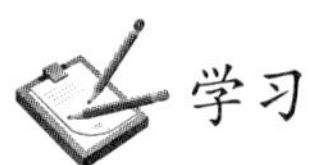
学习

Detection of small low-contrast objects was significantly easier using a masked viewbox with high luminance than using a regular unmasked viewbox. When a regular viewbox (approximately 3 000 nits) was used masking had a more significant effect on films with high optical densities than on films with low optical densities. Brighter, masked viewbox improved detection on films with higher optical densities.

利用遮蔽高亮度观片灯诊断小的低对比物显著易于常规未遮蔽观片灯。当常规观片灯（约 3 000 nits）遮蔽时，对于高光学密度照片比低光学密度照片更具有显著作用。高亮度遮蔽观片灯提高了高光学密度照片的诊断力。

nit [nit] *n*. 尼特（表面亮度单位）　　high optical densities 高光学密度

low optical densities 低光学密度

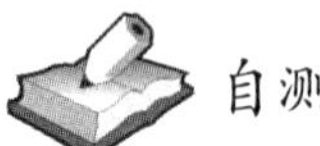
自测

Dose measurements with a chest phantom showed a dose reduction of approximately 50% with the digital radiography system compared with the film-screen radiography system. The image quality and the visibility of all but one anatomic structure of the images obtained with the digital flat-panel detector system were rated significantly superior ($P \leqslant 0.000\ 3$) to those obtained with the conventional film-screen radiography system.

答案

用胸部体模进行剂量测试显示，数字 X 线摄影系统相对于屏 - 片 X 线摄影系统剂量下降大约 50%。数字平板探测器系统所获得的影像的所有解剖结构（除 1 个外）的影像质量和可见度显著优于传统屏 - 片 X 线摄影系统获得的影像 ($P \leqslant 0.000\ 3$)。

all but 除了

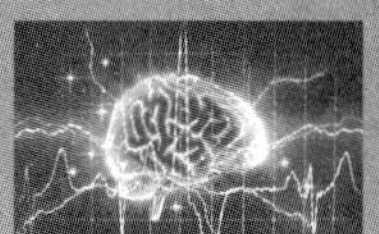

第 26 天

学习

The mean area under the ROC curves increased from 0.89 to 0.98 with the temporal subtraction images. When the paired digitized previous and current chest radiographs were viewed in conjunction with the temporal subtraction images, a significant improvement in detection of new abnormalities was achieved (P = 0.000 04), whereas the mean interpretation time was reduced by 19.3% (from 52 to 42 seconds, including the time to record the score and to move to the next case, P = 0.001 9).

采用时间减影图像 ROC 曲线下的平均面积从 0.89 增加到 0.98。当观察先前配对数字与当前胸部 X 线照片及时间减影图像时，发现新的异常能力得到显著提高（P=0.000 04），而平均判读时间下降 19.3%（从 52 s 降到 42 s，包括记分时间和换片时间，P=0.001 9）。

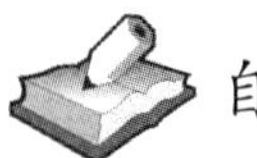

自测

No statistically significant differences were found in the area under the receiver operating characteristic curve for detecting urinary calculi or in the interpreting times between soft-copy and hard-copy images; the mean areas under the receiver operating characteristic curve of hard-copy images, soft-copy images displayed on an LCD monitor, and soft-copy images displayed on a high-resolution video monitor were 0.579, 0.610, and 0.732, respectively. However, soft-copy images showed relatively improved diagnostic accuracy among less experienced radiologists ($P < 0.05$).

答案

诊断尿路结石及判读时间上，软拷贝图像与硬拷贝图像之间其受试者作业特性曲线下的面积无显著统计学差异，硬拷贝图像、在 LCD 显示器上显示的软拷贝图像、在高分辨率图像显示器上显示的软拷贝图像的受试者作业特性曲线下的平均面积分别为 0.579、0.610、0.732。但是，缺乏经验的放射学家的软拷贝影像显示诊断精确性相对改善 ($P < 0.05$)。

no statistically significant differences 无显著统计学差异

the interpreting time 判读时间

a high-resolution video monitor 高分辨率图像显示器

第 27 天

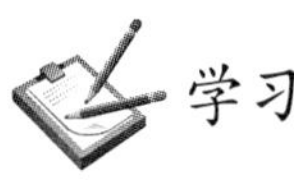

学习

表达研究结果的常用句式如下：

...increased (rise, raise) by 50%... ……增加了 50%……

...a 30% reduction (decrease, reduce, lower) in...was observed ……观察到降低 30%……

...resulted in a marked increase in... ……导致……明显增高

...was lowered from...to... ……从……下降到……

There was a significant linear correlation between...and... ……与……有显著的线性关系

...showed no strong correlation between...and... ……显示……与……无密切相关性

...correlated positively with... ……与……呈正相关

A negative correlation was found between...and... 发现……与……呈负相关

No statistical differences were observed between...and... ……与……之间未见统计学差异

...was closely related to... ……与……密切相关

...demonstrated a significant improvement in... ……方面呈明显改善

四、结 论

结论是根据结果所推出的论断及作者观点,往往采用概括性语言具体点出答案,有画龙点睛之作用。通常也可只用一句话表述。

第 28 天

Invasive breast cancer detection by mammography may be improved through attention to correct positioning.

通过正确的摄影定位可以改善乳腺 X 线摄影对侵袭性乳腺癌的诊断。

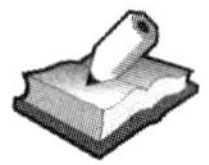

The temporal subtraction technique can significantly improve sensitivity and specificity for detection of interval change in chest radiographs.

时间减影技术能显著地改善胸部 X 线照片中间隔性改变的诊断灵敏度与特异性。

sensitivity [sensə'tivəti] *n.* 灵敏(度、性)　　specificity [ˌspesi'fisəti] *n.* 特异性

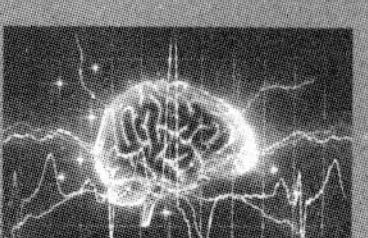

第 29 天

学习

Better detection of small low-contrast objects results when mammographic images are masked and viewed on high-luminance viewbox than when a regular unmasked viewbox is used.

乳腺 X 线照片采用遮蔽高亮度观片灯显示图像比使用常规未遮蔽观片灯更能较好地发现小的低对比物。

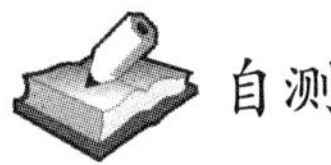

自测

The diagnostic performance of the new large-area silicon flat-panel detector is equivalent or superior to that of the conventional screen-film system for clinical chest imaging and can replace conventional radiography systems.

答案

对于临床胸部成像，新的大面积硅平板探测器的诊断性能等同于或优于传统屏 - 片的诊断性能，且可以替代传统 X 线摄影系统。

superior [sju(:)'piəriə] *a.* 上等的，在上的，占优的

be superior in 在……方面占优势，be superior to 优于、胜过

be superior to M in N　在 N 方面比 M 好　　rise superior to 超越

注：that 替代了 diagnostic performance，注意在比较句中，要同等东西进行比较，这个 that 万万不可省略。

第 30 天

学习

Use of flat-panel digital imagers based on the cesium iodide-amorphous silicon technique allows a considerable dose reduction during routine chest radiography without loss of image quality.

采用基于碘化铯非晶硅技术的平板数字成像仪进行常规胸部 X 线摄影，在不影响影像质量的同时可减少相当多的剂量。

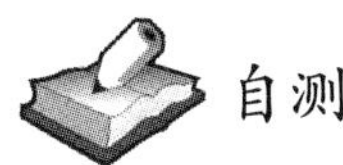

自测

Subjective visibility of normal anatomy of the hands and feet using selenium-based digital radiography was similar to that achieved using conventional film-screen radiography.

答案

采用以硒为基础的数字 X 线摄影，手和足的正常解剖的主观显示能力与采用传统屏 - 片 X 线摄影所获得的相似。

similar ['similə] *a.* 相似的　　be similar to 与……相似

in a similar way to 与……相似的方式　　somewhat similar to 有点类似于

第 31 天

学习

The image quality and visibility of anatomic structures on the images obtained by the flat-panel detector system were perceived as equal or superior to the images from conventional film-screen chest radiography. This was true even though the radiation dose was reduced approximately 50% with the digital flat-panel detector system.

采用平板探测系统获得的图像在影像质量和解剖结构的可见度上等同于或优于传统屏 - 片胸部 X 线摄影所获得的影像，甚至当数字平板探测器系统降低 50% 的放射剂量时也如此。

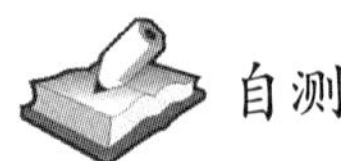
自测

For detecting urinary calculi, soft-copy images offered a diagnostic accuracy similar to or slightly more accurate than that of hard-copy images obtained in a laser-printed film-based environment. The diagnostic performance with soft-copy images viewed on an LCD monitor was comparable to that of soft-copy images viewed on a high-resolution video monitor.

答案

对于诊断尿路结石，软拷贝影像所提供的诊断精确性类似或稍高于以胶片为基础的激光打印所获得的硬拷贝图像。在 LCD 显示器上显示的软拷贝影像的诊断性能可以与在高分辨率图像显示器上显示的软拷贝图像相比。

environment [in'vaiərənmənt] *n.* 周围环境　　laser-printed 激光打印

注：obtained 过去分词作定语，也可改作 which are obtained。

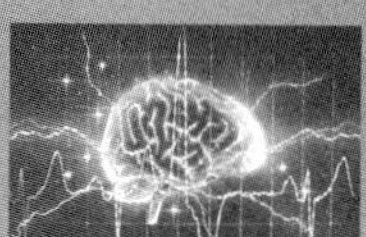

第 32 天

学习

In summary,our results show the potential of dual energy subtraction(DES) to improve computer-aided detection(CAD) sensitivity on certain subtle lung cancer lesions,and the decrease in CAD false-positive marks with DES should improve reader performance and radiologist acceptance of CAD technology. A rigorous reader study is planned to further evaluate the role and relative contributions of DES and chest CAD.

总之,我们的结果显示 DES 有提高 CAD 在某些微小肺癌病变的灵敏度上的潜能,CAD 假阳性标记降低与 DES 一起可提高判读仪的性能,以及提高放射学家对 CAD 技术的认可度。缜密的判读仪研究计划进一步评价 DES 和胸部 CAD 的角色及相关作用。

DES,dual energy subtraction 的缩写,双能量减影。

CAD,computer-aided detection 的缩写,计算机辅助检测。

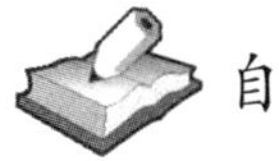

自测

水平干预——如随着放射学引导的操作流程、安全训练计划、防错训练和经验 - 教训交流计划——能成功地提高放射科安全文化及其性能。

答案

Horizontal interventions—such as operational rounds with radiology leadership,safety coach programs,error prevention training,and a lessons-learned communication program—can successfully improve the safety culture and performance in radiology.

第 33 天

学习

Because the total measured radiation dose is 32% greater from a single combination helical HRCT scan of the chest versus separate standard helical plus axial HRCT scans,helical HRCT is not a clinically advisable technique.

因为胸部单次结合螺旋高分辨率 CT 扫描,比独立标准螺旋加轴位高分辨率 CT 扫描的整体测试的放射剂量高 32%,所以螺旋高分辨率 CT 不是一种可推荐的临床技术。

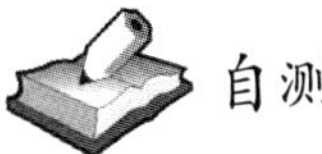

急诊科少部分患者 (1.9%) 进行了多次或是重复成像的颈部、胸部、腹部或骨盆的高累积率的 CT 检查。总的来讲,这少部分患者累积 CT 辐射曝光使之加剧了患癌症的风险。

A small proportion(1.9%) of emergency department patients undergoing CT of the neck,chest,abdomen,or pelvis have high cumulative rates of multiple or repeat imaging. Collectively,this patient subgroup may have a heightened risk of developing cancer from cumulative CT radiation exposure.

第 34 天

There were no significant differences between the 100% examinations and the 50% and 25% examinations for the detection of calculi greater than 3 mm.

对于 3 mm 以上结石的检查,在 100%、50%、25% 检查之间无显著性差异。

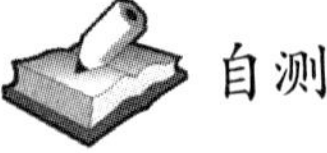

前瞻性成像采用容积扫描长度 120 ~ 140 mm 在临床实践中是可行的。在其他扫描参数不变的情况下,有效辐射剂量显著减少,从而使之成为富有吸引力的成像策略。

Prospective imaging with a volume scan length of 120—140 mm is feasible in clinical practice. Marked reduction in effective radiation dose without alteration of other scan parameters was achieved,making this an attractive imaging strategy.

第 35 天

表达作者结论的常用句式如下:

It was found that... 发现……

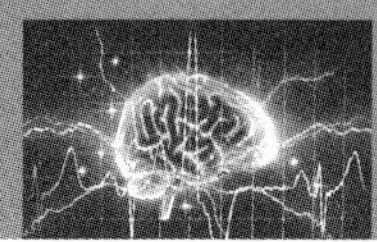

It was observed that... 观察到……

These results suggest that... 结果提示……

These findings indicate that... 这些发现表明……

Our observations confirm that... 我们的观察证实……

We conclude that... 我们的结论是……

We suggest that... 我们建议……

We believe that... 我们认为……

It is concluded that... 结论是……

It is suggested that... 建议……

It is recommended that... 建议……

It is estimated that... 估计……

From this study, we conclude that... 根据此项研究，我们的结论是……

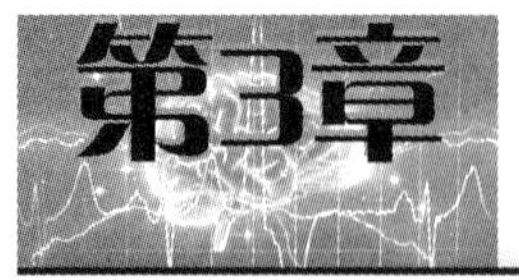

第3章 关键词（Key words）

为了让读者对全文或科研项目有一个大致的了解，通常采用能够代表其主题的关键词引导读者，也便于读者通过关键词作为索引（index terms）查找相关文献。有时为了更能确切地查找，或是便于读者理解，采用2个或2个以上关键词成为一组加以概括、辨析、理解、查找，通常为3～10组，位置分别位于摘要的下方。

第36天

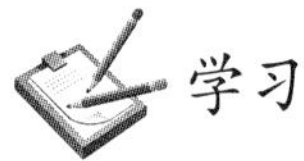

学习

1. Diagnostic radiology
   Lung nodule
   Receiver operating characteristic curve(ROC)
   X线诊断
   肺结节
   受试者作业特性曲线
2. Radiography
   Digital
   Thorax
   X线摄影
   数字
   胸部

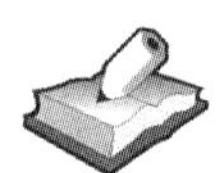

自测

1. 双能量减影
   数字X线摄影

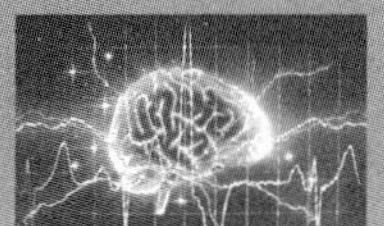

计算机辅助诊断

肺结节

2. 洗片机

胶片

质量控制

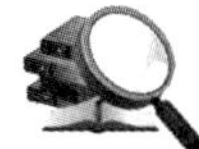

答案

1. Dual energy subtraction

Digital radiography

Computer-aided detection

Pulmonary nodules

2. Processor

Film

Quality control

第 37 天

学习

1. Wrist

Arthrography

Injuries

腕关节

关节造影

损伤

arthrography [ɑː'θrɔgrəfi] *n.* 关节造影

2. Quality control

Quality improvement

Quality assurance

Cardiopulmonary radiology

质量控制

质量改善

质量保证

心肺 X 线摄影

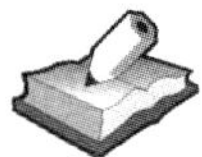

自测

1. 计算机断层扫描
   放射剂量
   成像参数
   临床协议
2. 多排探测器 CT
   容积分析
   工作站

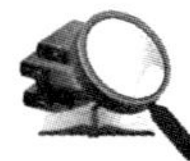

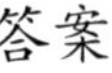

答案

1. Computed tomography
   Radiation dose
   Imaging parameters
   Clinical protocols
2. MDCT
   Volumetric analysis
   Workstation

第 38 天

学习

1. CT
   Radiation dose
   Radiation practice
   Radiation risks
   计算机断层扫描
   放射剂量
   放射实践
   放射风险
2. Coronary CT angiography
   Image quality
   Radiation dose
   Tube voltage

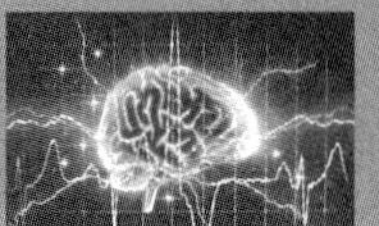

冠状动脉 CT 血管造影
图像质量
放射剂量
管电压

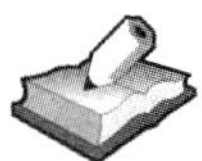

自测

1. 颅脑解剖
   颅脑磁共振
   颅脑 CT
2. 放射诊断
   数字 X 线摄影
   乳腺 X 线摄影
   影像后处理
3. 乳腺 X 线摄影
   质量保证
   图像，伪影

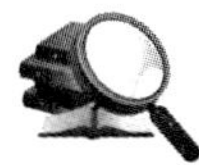

答案

1. Brain anatomy
   Brain MR
   Brain CT
2. Diagnostic radiology
   Digital radiography
   Mammography radiography
   Image processing
3. Breast radiography
   Quality assurance
   Images, artifact

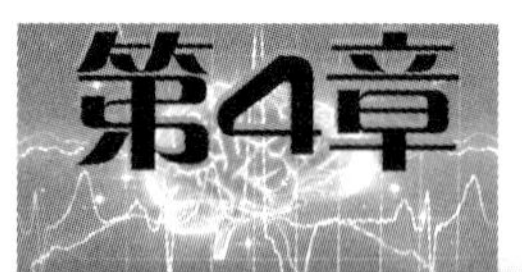

第4章 引言（Introduction）

引言为文章的开头，概括性地回顾历史，阐述学术现状、存在的不足，指明作者所要研究、探讨的问题，有时也称背景。

在引言阐述中，作者要明确表达研究的动机、研究的前提、研究的依据、研究的任务、研究的范围，打算通过什么途径，在哪个层次上开展研究，提出拟解决的关键性问题，甚至还可以概括其学术地位、实际与理论意义研究的迫切性和必要性。

总之，对引言的描述应当明确、具体、针对性强，应开门见山，且不宜过长，一般 100 ~ 200 字即可。

一、 概述学术现状

应用精练的语言概括性地回顾历史，阐述学术现状、存在的问题。

第 39 天

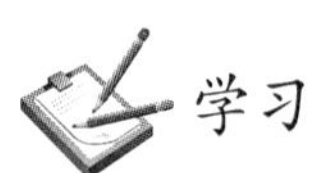

学习

Although computed radiography (CR) images are acquired using conventional imaging geometry, grids, and X-ray tables and tubes, certain aspects of the technology produce artifacts. The imaging plate, the plate reader, image processing and operator errors may all contribute to the artifacts. Knowledge of how each of these factors contributes artifacts to the imaging process will assist in troubleshooting.

虽然利用传统的几何学成像原理、滤线栅、X 线控制台及 X 线管可获得计算机 X 线摄影（computed radiography，CR）图像，但是该技术在运用过程中会产生伪影。成像板、成像板阅读器、影像处理及操作者失误都有可能产生伪影。了解成像过程中这些因素是如何导致伪影的产生将有助于解决难题。

geometry [dʒi'ɔmitri] *n.* 几何学　　grid 滤线栅

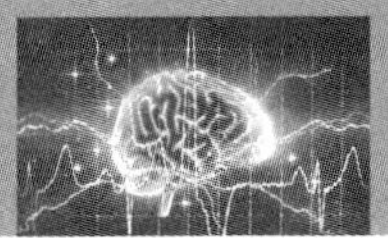

tube[tju:b] *n*. 球管
aspect['æspekt] *n*.(问题、事物等的)方面
imaging plate 成像板,简称 IP
reader['ri:də] *n*. 阅读器
process['prəuses　'prɔses] *vt*. 加工、处理
contribute to 产生
factor['fæktə] *n*. 因素、原因
assist in doing sth.(或 assist sb. with sth.,或 assist to do sth.)有助于
troubleshoot['trʌblʃu:t] 消除缺陷、发现缺点

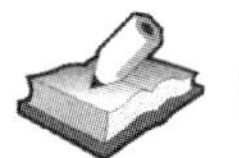
自测

胸部 X 线摄影要求较高,因为人体组织的密度范围广,因而需要特殊技术处理。传统屏 - 片系统的主要优势是高空间分辨率、大面积范围内良好的均一性、高灵敏度、易操作性及低成本,但胶片曝光宽容度窄是这些系统的局限。采用大宽容度胶片及高千伏技术可以在一定程度上克服这个问题。

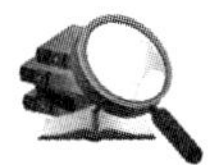
答案

Chest radiology is highly demanding, because there are special technical requirements that result from the wide range of tissue densities. The main advantages of conventional screen-film systems are high spatial resolution, good uniformity over a large area, high sensitivity, easy handling, and low cost, but these systems are limited by the small exposure range of the film. Using wide-latitude film and performing the technique at a high kilovoltage are suitable to overcome this problem to a certain extent.

advantage[əd'vɑ:ntidʒ] *n*. 优势、有利条件
spatial resolution 空间分辨率
handling *n*. 操作
limited['limitid] *a*. 有限的
high kilovoltage 高千伏
result from 由……引起
suitable['sju:təbl] *a*. 合适的、适宜的、适当的
result in 导致
uniformity[ˌju:ni'fɔ:məti] *n*. 均匀(性、度)

第 40 天

学习

Digital system provides a wide dynamic range, which is preferable in chest imaging. The first step in digital chest radiology was the use of storage phosphor plates, which provide images of equivalent quality compared with those of conventional screen-film system. However, a higher radiation dose is needed to achieve a similar contrast resolution.

数字系统提供了一个宽广的动态范围,这尤其适用于胸部成像。数字胸部 X 线摄影的

第一步是使用储存荧光板,它能够生成质量足以与传统屏 - 片系统相媲美的影像。然而,为了达到相似的对比分辨率,需要较高的放射剂量。

a wide dynamic range 宽的动态范围　　storage phosphor plate 存储荧光板
equivalent [i'kwivələnt] *a.* 相同的、相当的、等价的、等效的
(as) compared with 与……比较　　contrast resolution 对比分辨率

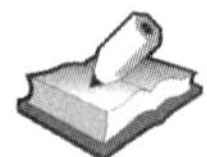
自测

许多厂商正在研究使用固态数字探测器进行 X 线摄影。这些数字探测器由一可将 X 线转换成光或电子电荷的物质层构成。这种光或电子电荷被半导体元素(判读层)转换成数字数据。X 线转换层与判读层构造成一种物理器件,消除了屏 - 片形式及计算机 X 线摄影所必需的判读或显影装置分离。

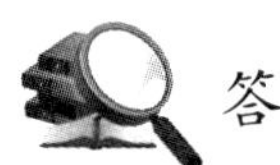
答案

Several manufacturers are researching solid-state digital detectors for radiography. These digital detectors consist of a layer of material that converts X rays to light or electric charges. The light or electric charges are converted into digital data by arrays of semiconductor elements (readout layer). One physical device constructed by the X-ray conversion layer and the readout layer eliminates the need for a separate readout or development device, as necessary for film-screen and computed radiography.

solid-state *a.* 固态的、硬的　　convert M to(into) N　把 M 转变成 N
electric charge 电子电荷　　array [ə'rei] *n.* 排、列
semiconductor element 半导体元素　　readout layer 判读层
eliminate [i'limineit] *vt.* 消除　　development [di'veləpmənt] *n.* 显影、冲洗
separate ['sepəreit] *a.v.* 分离

第 41 天

学习

Recently, direct-readout radiography system was developed. The systems are flat-panel X-ray detectors with either an integrated charge-coupled device or an integrated thin-film transistor (TFT) readout mechanism. Various types of TFT detectors have been studied. All detectors are based on amorphous silicon TFT technology, but each is combined with different types of converter arrays, which convert X-ray beams to electric charges directly or indirectly.

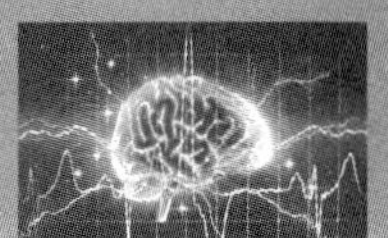

近来，直接判读 X 线影像的系统已研制。这些系统是平板 X 线探测器附加集成电子耦合器件或集成电路薄膜晶体管（thin-film transistor, TFT）判读仪。人们已研究了各种类型的 TFT 探测器。所有探测器均基于非晶硅 TFT 技术，但每一种都是由不同类型转换器排列组合而成，正是这些不同的排列组合将 X 线直接或间接地转换成电子电荷。

direct-readout radiography system 直接判读 X 线摄影系统

flat-panel X-ray detector 平板 X 线探测器

either...or... 或者……或者，不论……还是

integrate ['intigreit] *vt.* 使结合；*vi.*（与……）结合起来（with）

charge-coupled device 电子耦合器件，简称 CCD

thin-film transistor 薄膜晶体管

converter *n.* 转换器

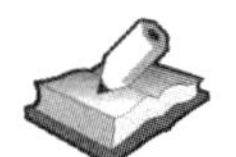

自测

固态数字 X 线捕捉系统相比屏 - 片系统及计算机 X 线摄影有许多潜在的优势。固态数字系统的优势包括把显影或判读影像的装置合二为一，患者定位及曝光条件可即时反馈给技师，并快速获得影像，增加患者流量，加快电子影像传输及电子影像显示。然而，全视野（35 cm × 43 cm 或更大）固体探测器必须显示出与传统屏 - 片 X 线摄影相等的影像质量及诊断的精确性，才能使此技术被广为接受。

答案

Solid-state digital X-ray capture system has several potential advantages over film-screen system and computed radiography. The advantages of solid-state digital system include elimination of a separate device to develop or read the image, immediate feedback to the technologists on patient positioning and exposure, faster availability of the image, increased patient throughput, electronic image transmission, and electronic image display. However, full-field (35 cm × 43 cm or larger) solid-state detectors need to show equivalent image quality and diagnostic accuracy to those of conventional film-screen radiography for this technology to be accepted.

feedback ['fi:dbæk] *n.* 反馈

technologist　*n.* 技术人员（专家）

exposure [iks'pəuʒə] *n.* 曝光、照射

throughput [θru:'put] *n.* 通过量、吞吐量

transmission [trænz'miʃən] *n.* 传输、发送

display [dis'plei] *vt.* 显示、呈现

equivalent [i'kwivələnt] *a.* 相等的、等价的

第 42 天

学习

Chest radiography plays an essential role in the diagnosis of thoracic disease and is the most frequently performed radiologic examination in the United States. Since the discovery of X rays more than a century ago, advances in technology have yielded numerous improvements in thoracic imaging. Evolutionary progress in film-based imaging has led to the development of excellent screen-film systems specifically designed for chest radiography. In addition, recent revolutionary advances in electronic and computer technology have enabled the development of digital image receptor and display, creating new opportunities in the practice of diagnostic imaging.

胸部 X 线摄影在胸部疾病的诊断方面发挥着必不可少的作用，且在美国放射学检查中运用频率最高。自从一个多世纪前发现 X 线以来，该技术的进展，在胸部成像方面已经取得了很大的提高。在以胶片为基础的成像方面所取得的长足进步已经导致特别为胸部 X 线摄影而设计的优质屏 - 片系统的开发。此外，近来在电子、计算机技术方面所取得的革命性进展已经使数字影像接收器和显示器研制成为可能，并在影像诊断的实践中创造新的机遇。

play an essential role 起着必不可少的作用

thoracic [θɔ:'ræsik] *a.* 胸的

disease [di'zi:z] *n.* 疾病

numerous ['nju:mərəs] *a.* 为数众多的

opportunity [ˌɔpə'tju:nəti] *n.* 机会

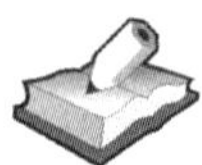

自测

基于碘化铯（cesium iodide，CsI）和非晶硅（amorphous silicon，a-Si）的敏感基质平板 X 摄影探测器可以提供高空间分辨率、高对比分辨率的数字 X 线照片，这种探测器还具有降低 X 线剂量的潜能。以前绝大多数实验系统和比较小的探测器原型的试验和临床研究显示：这种技术比传统屏 - 片系统优秀。

答案

Active matrix flat-panel radiography detector based on cesium iodide and amorphous silicon provides digital radiographs with high spatial and contrast resolution and has the potential to allow a reduction in radiation dose. Previous experimental and clinical studies, mostly with experimental system and detector prototype of limited size, have shown excellent results compared with conventional film-screen system.

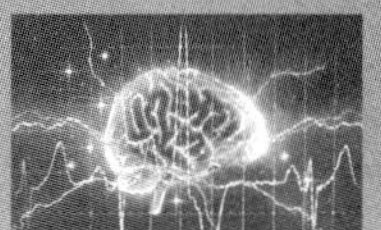

第 43 天

学习

Digital X-ray detector based on the cesium iodide (CsI) and amorphous silicon (a-Si) technique provides wide exposure latitude and high contrast resolution with a detective quantum efficiency superior to that of conventional and storage phosphor radiography. Favorable results in detectability of simulated pulmonary lesions have been reported for an experimental, flat-panel CsI/a-Si detector of limited size compared with the results obtained using screen-film radiography.

基于碘化铯（cesium iodide，CsI）和非晶体硅（amorphous silicon，a-Si）技术的数字 X 线探测器提供较广的曝光宽容度和高对比分辨率，量子检出效率（detective quantum efficiency，DQE）优于传统和存储荧光 X 线摄影。在仿真肺部病变的探测能力中，用较小的平板 CsI/a-Si 探测器与用屏 - 片 X 线摄影所获得的结果进行试验比较，已有了良好的结果。

detective quantum efficiency 量子检出效率，简称 DQE

simulate ['simjuleit] *vt.* 模拟、仿真、假装　　pulmonary ['pʌlmənəri] *a.* 肺的

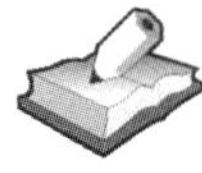

自测

目前，基于非晶硒探测器的新一代数字 X 线摄影系统正在涌现。基于硒的探测器原先用于乳腺 X 线摄影照片以外的系统，最近它和电子判读装置结合生成为数字 X 线摄影系统高效率、低噪声的接收器。非晶硒或 a-Se 已经被发现具有优质量子检出效率，这说明通过它生成的影像具有等同于或超过传统胶片的影像质量的潜能。针对此项的临床和实验研究的发现为这些预测提供了数据支持。

答案

A new generation of digital radiography system based on amorphous selenium detector is now emerging. Originally used in xenoradiographic system for mammography, selenium-based detector has recently been coupled with electronic readout mechanisms to create highly efficient, low-noise receptor for digital radiography system. Amorphous selenium, or a-Se, has been found to have excellent detective quantum efficiency, which would suggest the potential for image quality that equals or exceeds that of conventional film. Findings in initial clinical and laboratory studies provided data support for these predictions.

emerge [i'mə:dʒ] *vi.* 浮现、出现、形成　　couple ['kʌpl] *vt.* 连接、结合、使耦合

mechanism ['mekənizəm] *n.* 机械、装置　　low-noise receptor 低噪声接收器

prediction [pri'dikʃən] *n.* 预言、预告

第 44 天

学习

In addition to the excellent X-ray detection capabilities of amorphous selenium, another less advantageous characteristic property of this material also exists: The ability of selenium to capture a radiographic image can be noticeably altered immediately after exposure to a high-intensity X-ray source. Specifically, when a portion of the selenium detector is exposed to direct radiation (as often occurs in chest radiography) and additional radiographs are obtained soon thereafter, a silhouette of the first radiographic image can appear in the subsequent images until such time when the selenium has recovered from the initial exposure. In clinical practice, this so-called "memory" or "ghost" artifact can arise when a lateral chest radiograph is obtained (which usually exposes pant of the selenium receptor to direct, high-intensity radiation) and then, soon thereafter, a posteroanterior chest radiograph is obtained. In this case, the silhouette of the lateral chest radiograph sometimes can be seen superimposed on the posteroanterior image.

非晶硒除具有优秀的 X 线探测能力的优势外，还有另一个稍逊一些的本质特性：当高强度 X 线照射硒后，它捕捉 X 线影像的能力会立即发生显著的改变。尤其是当一部分硒探测器被射线直接照射（常见于胸部 X 线摄影），并且稍后又做其他 X 线摄影时，首次 X 线摄影的影像轮廓能显示在后面的影像上，直到硒从首次曝光后得到恢复时才消失。临床实践中，在摄取侧位胸部 X 线摄影（取侧位时常使用高强度射线直接照射部分硒接收器）并随后摄取后前位胸部 X 线摄影时，会出现这个所谓的"记忆"或"幻影"伪影。在这种情况下，有时能看到侧位胸部 X 线摄影的轮廓重叠在后前位影像上。

in addition to 除……之外

characteristic [ˌkæriktə'ristik] *n.* 特征、性能

property ['prɔpəti] *n.* 性质、特性　　exist [ig'zist] *vi.* 存在、有

capture ['kæptʃə] *vt.* 捕捉

radiographic [ˌreidiəu'græfik] *a.*X 线照相的

noticeably *ad.* 引人注意地、显著地　　alter ['ɔ:ltə] *v.* 改变、变更

intensity [in'tensiti] *n.* 强度　　source [sɔ:s] *n.* 源、出处

radiograph [ˌreidiəugrɑ:f] X 线照相

silhouette [ˌsilu'et] *n.* 轮廓、侧面影像、剪影

subsequent ['sʌbsikwənt] *a.* 后来的　　pant [pænt] *n.* 气喘、心跳

superimpose ['sju:pərim'pəuz] *vt.* 把……放在另一物的上面、附加

as often occurs 经常发生

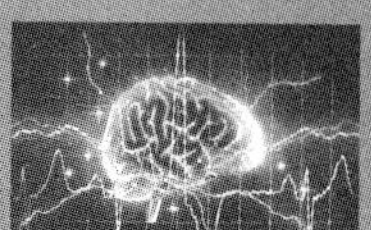

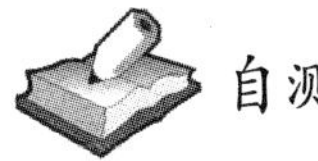

自测

硒记忆伪影被认为是由影像接收器的有效饱和度所引起的，其原因是在非晶硒层中，由于 X 线照射，产生了局部空间大范围充电及所谓的“深部空穴陷阱”现象。这个记忆作用会在几分钟后消退，取决于 X 线的强度和硒探测器的内部结构。

答案

The selenium memory artifact is known to result from effective saturation of the image receptor owing to the X-ray-induced generation of local bulk space charge and so-called “deep hole traps” in the amorphous selenium layer. How many minutes will be taken for the memory effect to dissipate depends on the X-ray intensity and the composition of the selenium detector.

be known to 为……所知

saturation [ˌsætʃə'reiʃn] *n.* 饱和

induce [in'dju:s] *vt.* 诱发、引起、导致

generation [dʒenə'reiʃən] *n.* 产生、引起

bulk [bʌlk] *n.* 大量、容量

trap [træp] *n.* 陷阱

dissipate ['disipeit] *v.* 消散、消除

composition [kɔmpə'ziʃən] *n.* 组成、成分、构成、合成

第 45 天

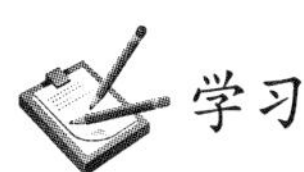

学习

Currently, only one selenium-based digital radiography system is commercially available. However, recent reports suggest that additional selenium-based digital system including a flat-panel and “direct radiography” cassette may soon become commercially available. Therefore, it is important for radiologists to recognize the potential to create memory artifacts in the system of this type.

目前，市场上只有一种基于硒的数字 X 线摄影系统。然而，近来报道显示另一种装有一个平面控制面板和可“直接 X 线摄影”暗盒的基于硒的数字系统或许不久会上市。因此，对于放射从业人员来说，认识到此类系统会生成潜在的记忆伪影非常重要。

cassette [kæ'set] *n.* 暗盒

commercially available 用于商业用途

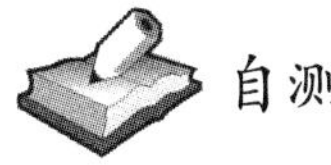

自测

在临床实践中，通常胸部 X 线照片的判读是对照同一患者以前获得的 X 线照片。在我们的研究所中，大约 80% 的胸部 X 线照片与先前的 X 线检查相对照判读。对照判读可帮助

放射学家识别异常并确定其临床意义，但重要的、细微的间隔性改变仅在回顾性判读时才被识别。在数字X线照片的情况下，能从当前的X线照片减去先前的X线照片产生的时间减影图像，以增强间隔性改变的区域。患者定位的不同影响时间减影图像的质量，但在减影前用几何卷积的方法来改进影像重合度，可部分克服这个缺点。

答案

In clinical practice, chest radiographs are commonly interpreted in comparison with previous radiographs obtained in the same patient. In our institution, approximately 80% of chest radiographs are interpreted side by side with previous examinations. Such comparison reading helps radiologists identify abnormalities and determine their clinical importance, but important interval changes may be subtle and identified only in retrospect. In the case of digital radiographs, it is possible to register and subtract the temporal subtraction image of the previous radiograph from the current one to enhance the area of interval change. The quality of the temporal subtraction image is considerably affected by variations in patient positioning, but this limitation can be partially overcome by geometrically warping one of the images to improve registration before subtraction.

previous ['pri:vjəs] *a.* 早先的、以前的

institution [ˌinsti'tju:ʃn] *n.* 学校、研究所

approximately [ə'prɔksimitli] *ad.* 近似地、大致

identify [ai'dentifai] *v.* 识别、辨认

subtle ['sʌtl] *a.* 微妙的、细微的

retrospect ['retrəspekt] *n.* 回顾、追溯

register ['redʒistə] *n.* 记录

subtract [səb'trækt] *v.* 减去；subtraction [səb'trækʃən] *n.* 减去

current ['kʌrənt] *a.* 当前的

temporal ['tempərəl] *a.* 瞬时的、短暂的

enhance [in'hɑ:ns] *vt.* 增强

side by side 并排地、一起

interval ['intəvəl] *n.* 间隔

第 46 天

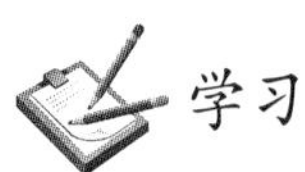

学习

For most mechanical helical CT scanners, scan times are 1 sec per 360° gantry rotation or 1 sec per revolution (spr), except for incomplete quick scan or half-scan data acquisitions and reconstruction algorithms. The limitations of rapid acquisition by helical CT scanners are

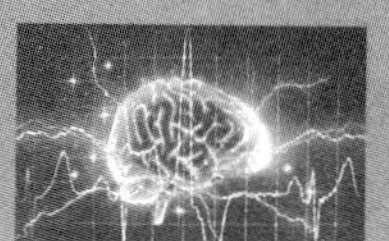

the increased demands on X-ray generators, X-ray tubes, and cooling mechanisms. Region (Z-axis) coverage per scan time is a compromise between collimation, pitch, and X-ray tube output. Technical advances have allowed an even further reduction of scan time to 0.75 spr. The advantages of faster scanning include longer Z-axis coverage for an equivalent duration of exposure or equivalent Z-axis coverage with thinner collimation. However, reduced image quality and decreased spatial resolution are possible because of a reduced number of projections. Lower mAs values at equivalent amperage settings may result in increased image noise.

对于大多数机械螺旋 CT 扫描机来说,除了不完全快速扫描或半扫描数据采集和重建算法外,扫描时间采用机架每旋转 360° 为 1 s 或 1 spr。螺旋 CT 扫描机快速采集数据的局限之处是对 X 线发生器、X 线管和冷却装置有较高的要求。每次扫描时间范围的区域(Z 轴)应兼顾准直器、螺距和 X 线管的输出。技术的提高已进一步将扫描时间减少至 0.75 spr。快速扫描的优点包括对于相同的曝光时间有较长 Z 轴区域或对于同样 Z 轴区域有较薄的准直。尽管如此,减少投影的数目可能会降低影像质量和空间分辨率。在相同安培数情况下,低毫安秒会导致影像噪声增加。

gantry ['gæntri] *n.* 机架

revolution [revə'lu:ʃən] *n.* 转动

generator ['dʒenəreitə] *n.* 发生器

output ['autput] *n.* 效率、输出量、功率

noise [nɔiz] *n.* 噪声

amperage ['æmpəridʒ] *n.* 安培数、电流量、电流强度

rotation [rəu'teiʃn] *n.* 旋转

algorithm ['ælgəriðəm] *n.* 算法

collimation [kɔli'meiʃən] *n.* 准直

duration [djuə'reiʃən] *n.* 持续

自测

在众多检查中,CT 在评价腕部方面有一个已被公认的作用,包括隐蔽型或复合型骨折的急性外伤、骨折愈合的评价和术后评价。腕部直接冠状 CT 成像因垂直诸多腕部关节面,从分辨率和判定容易两方面来说均优于轴位扫描。典型的用于直接冠状腕部成像的患者定位技术比常规 CT 成像进步了,后者要求患者保持几分钟不动。因为冠状扫描使需要覆盖腕部的 Z 轴层数减到最小,用窄的准直器 1 次 20 ~ 24 s 螺旋 CT 扫描就能完成,螺旋 CT 要求的短采集时间减少或消除层间的失准并适用于简化的患者定位。

答案

CT has an established role in evaluating the wrist in many applications, including acute trauma with occult or complex fractures, assessment of fracture healing, and postsurgical evaluation. Direct coronal CT imaging of the wrist produces slices perpendicular to the orientation of most carpal joints, providing advantages over axial acquisition both in resolution and in ease of interpretation. The patient-positioning techniques typically used for direct coronal wrist imaging

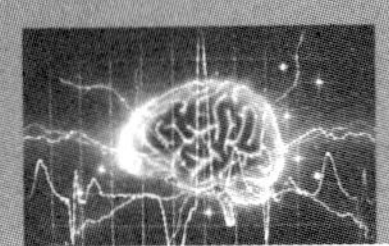

were developed to allow the patient to remain motionless for the several minutes required for conventional CT imaging. Because coronal acquisition minimizes the Z-axis distance needed to cover the wrist, it can be accomplished with a single 20—24 s helical CT scan even with narrow collimation. The short acquisition time required for helical CT minimizes or eliminates misregistration between slices and permits simplified patient positioning.

establish [is'tæbliʃ] *vt.* 建立、形成、产生、证实　　acute [ə'kju:t] *a.* 急性的
trauma ['trɔ:mə]（复数 traumas 或 traumata）*n.* 损伤、外伤、创伤
occult [ə'kʌlt] *a.* 隐的、难懂的
complex ['kɔmpleks] *a.* 复杂的
fracture ['fræktʃə] *n.* 骨折　　heal [hi:l] *v.* 治愈
coronal ['kɔrənl] *a.* 冠状的
perpendicular [pə:pən'dikjulə] 与……垂直的（to）
orientation [ɔ:rien'teiʃən] *n.* 定向的　　carpal ['ka:pl] *a.* 腕的
joint [dʒɔint] *n.* 关节　　axial ['æksiəl] *a.* 轴的
motionless ['məuʃnləs] *a.* 不动的、固定的、静止的
axis ['æksis]（复数 axes）*n.* 轴、中心线、枢椎
misregistration *n.* 配准不良

第 47 天

学习

Computed tomographic (CT) urography is a developing concept that combines portions of intravenous urography and CT into one examination, hence requiring only a single dose of intravenously administered iodinated contrast media. Intravenous urography and CT each have strengths and weaknesses in the evaluation of the urinary tract. CT is superior for the detection of urinary stone disease and for the evaluation of the renal parenchyma and adjacent structures and organs. Intravenous urography is better for evaluating the pyelocalyceal collecting system and ureters, because of the superior spatial resolution of radiography [≈ 4 line pairs per millimeter for screen-film radiography (S-F)] compared with that of CT (≈ 0.7 line pairs per millimeter for abdominal CT). Specifically, intravenous urography is considered superior for the delineation of calyceal and papillary anatomy, collecting ducts, mucosal detail, and small filling defects. In our experience, we have found that 10% of urinary tract abnormalities were depicted more clearly or appreciated only on S-F urographic images when compared with CT cross-sectional images. Hence, by combining the strengths of each study into one CT urographic examination, the urinary tract can be evaluated more thoroughly in a single session.

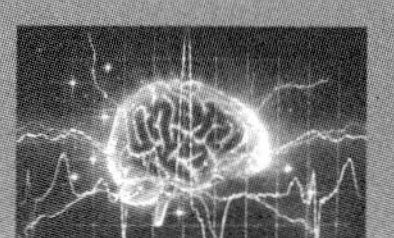

计算机断层扫描（computed tomographic, CT）尿路造影是一个发展中的概念，是把静脉尿路造影和 CT 组合起来应用到同一个检查中，因此，只需要单次静脉注射碘对比剂。静脉尿路造影和 CT 在尿路的评价方面各有利弊。对于尿结石的诊断、肾实质以及相邻结构和器官的评价上 CT 占优势。而对于评价肾盏收集系统和输尿管则静脉尿路造影较好，因为 X 线照片的空间分辨率［对于屏 - 片 X 线照片（screen-film, S-F）约为 4 线对 /mm］优于 CT 的空间分辨率（对于腹部 CT 约为 0.7 线对 /mm）。尤其认为静脉尿路造影对于肾盏和肾乳头解剖的描绘、收集管、黏膜细节以及小的充盈缺损具有优势。根据我们的经验，我们发现与 CT 横断影像相比尿路异常的 10% 仅在 S-F 尿路造影影像上被更清晰或正确地描绘。因此，将各种研究的优势结合到 CT 尿路造影检查中，使尿路能在一次检查中完全地被评价。

administer［əd'ministə］*vt.* 给予、用药
strength［streŋθ］*a.* 强度、力量、浓度
urinary［'juərinəri］*a.* 尿的、泌尿的
renal［'ri:nl］*a.* 肾的
adjacent［ə'dʒeisənt］*a.* 邻近的、毗连的
organ［'ɔ:gən］*n.* 器官
abdominal［æb'dɔminl］*a.* 腹部的
delineation［di'lini'eiʃn］*n.* 轮廓、描绘
calyceal［ˌkæli'siəl］*a.* 盏的
papillary［pə'piləri］*a.* 乳头的、乳头状的
mucosal *a.* 黏膜
cross-sectional image 横断面影像
iodinated contrast media 碘对比剂
weakness *n.* 虚弱
tract［trækt］*n.* 道
parenchyma［pə'reŋkimə］*n.* 实质
structure［'strʌktʃə］*n.* 结构
ureter［ju'ri:tə］*n.* 输尿管
pyelocalyceal 肾盏
duct［dʌkt］*n.* 导管
defect［di'fekt］*n.* 缺损、缺陷

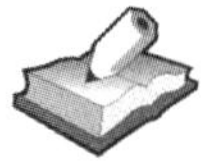

自测

16 排探测器 CT（computed tomographic, CT）技术的引入被认为是无创心脏成像的一大进步。尤其是其亚秒级的转速和窄的准直器解决了长久以来需要权衡扫描容积和层厚的弊端，并可以收集大量容积数据，使层厚重建到亚毫米级。但是，空间分辨率对 CT 心脏影像质量的影响比时间分辨率（获得每 1 幅横断图像所需时间）小。在心跳周期的任何阶段（回顾心电门控性技术）原则上可以同时采集成像及心电图资料，在扫描时对数据进行连续薄层重建。

答案

The introduction of 16-detector row computed tomographic (CT) technology is commonly regarded as a further step toward noninvasive CT cardiac imaging. Particularly, the combination of subsecond rotation and narrow collimation resolved the long-lasting trade-off between scanning volume and section thickness and enabled the acquisition of large scanning volume data sets, as well as reconstructed into sections of submillimeter thickness. Unfortunately, CT cardiac image quality is determined less on the basis of spatial resolution than on the basis of temporal resolution (ie, the time needed for acquisition of each transverse image). In principle, simultaneous acquisition of imaging and electrocardiographic data during scanning allows the reconstruction of continuous thin-section volume data sets during any phase of the cardiac cycle (retrospective electrocardiographic gating).

noninvasive [ˌnɔnin'veisiv] *a.* 非侵袭的　　cardiac imaging 心脏成像
trade-off *n.* 折中、权衡　　temporal resolution 时间分辨率

第 48 天

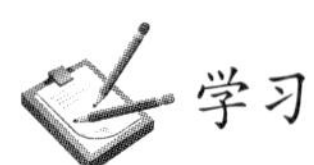

学习

Preferably, reconstruction of multi-detector row cardiac CT images is performed within middiastole, which commonly represents the longest and calmest period in the cardiac cycle. According to cardiac mechanics, however, it is the transition between end systole and early diastole that displays the least cardiac motion. This becomes apparent in patients with high heart rates when the diastole and, most important, the middiastole markedly decrease and finally fall short into the systole. Thus, from a physiologic point of view, an image reconstruction technique solely based on middiastole may not be the best strategy for delivering optimal image quality.

多排探测器 CT 最好是将重建图像置于心脏舒张中期，因为在心脏跳动周期中，这段时间是最长且相对平静的时期。根据心脏力学，心脏在收缩末期至舒张早期因心脏运动而能够显示的时间最小。尤其是在高心率患者中，心舒期缩短，并很快进入收缩期，这种现象就变得更为明显。因此，从生理角度看，图像重建技术完全基于心脏舒张中期未必是提供最佳图像质量的最好策略。

systole ['sistəli] *n.* 收缩期　　diastole [dai'æstəli] *n.* 舒张期
cardiac cyde 心脏周期

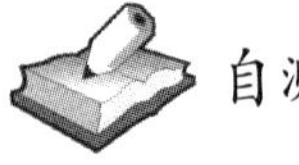

自测

在过去的几年里，空间分辨率和时间分辨率的提高致使高度狭窄病变的诊断图像质量更好、准确性更高。因此，16 层和 64 层 CT（computed tomographic，CT）具有改善高心率患者的图像质量和减少由于重度钙化引起的放射状伪影的潜力。研究发现，即使是 64 层 CT 有时 330 ms 的机架旋转速度和 0.4 mm^3 的空间各向同性分辨率，更高的不规则的心率仍然会引起图像质量的下降。还有，严重的钙化被认为与图像诊断正确率的降低有关联。

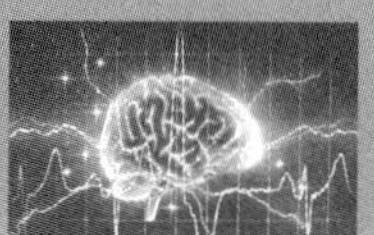

答案

In the past few years, advances in spatial and temporal resolution translated into better image quality and improved accuracy for the detection of high-grade stenosis. Thereby, 16-section and 64-section computed tomographic (CT) technology had the potential to extend acceptable image quality to higher heart rates and likewise reduce blooming artifacts related to heavy calcification. However, even with 64-section CT, with its superior gantry rotation speed of 330 ms and isotropic spatial resolution of 0.4 mm^3, elevated and irregular heartbeats were found to cause relevant degradation of image quality. Moreover, severe calcification has persistently been linked to a decrease in diagnostic accuracy.

stenosis [sti'nəusis] *n.* 狭窄；复数 stenoses

blooming ['blu:miŋ] *n.* 模糊现象、开花效应

isotropic [ˌaisə'trɔpik] *a.* 各向同性的

relevant ['relivənt] *a.* 相应的；be relevant to (with) 和……有关的

elevated ['eliveitid] *a.* 升高的

irregular heartbeat 不规则心率

persistent [pə'sistənt] *a.* 持久的

第 49 天

学习

Recently, a CT system equipped with two tubes and corresponding detectors in a 90° geometry has been designed and provides temporal resolution of approximately a quarter of its 330 ms gantry rotation time. This approach thus allows a temporal resolution of 83 ms, which is independent of the patient's heart rate and eliminates the need for dual-segment reconstruction algorithms. Results of pilot studies on cardiac applications of this dual-source CT system have been promising, and results of a feasibility study have shown excellent accuracy for detection of coronary artery disease in an unselected patient cohort. However, to date, effects of heart rate and heart rate variability on diagnostic accuracy have not been systematically assessed in a larger patient cohort to our knowledge.

最近，一套配备了 2 套 X 线管及其相对应的探测器交叉成 90° 的 CT 系统已研制成功，它可提供接近 1/4 330 ms 的时间分辨率。这一设备的时间分辨率即为 83 ms，这使其不依赖于患者的心率，并消除了对双扇区图像重建算法的需要。双源 CT 系统在心脏方面应用的前瞻性研究结果表明它是非常有前景的，其可行性研究的结果显示其在一组非特选患者的冠状动脉疾病的诊断中有极高的准确度。尽管如此，到目前为止，心率及心率变化对诊断精度的影响仍然没有通过大样本得到系统的评估。

corresponding *a.* 相当的、对应的、一致的

algorithm ['ælgəriðəm] *n.* 算法、规则系统

equip [i'kwip] *vt.* 装备 (equipped, equipping); equip M for N 装备 M 以便 N
dual-segment reconstruction algorithms 双扇区重建算法
cohort ['kəuhɔ:t] *n.* 一群　　pilot ['pailət] *a.* 先导的

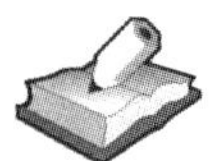 自测

正电子发射断层显像技术 (positron emission tomography, PET) 现今已被常规地应用于临床成像中。先前的研究表明：伴随着对光量子衰减的校正，用 PET 诊断人体深部病变的技术得到了完善。最近，不同的厂家引入 PET/ 计算机断层扫描 (computed tomography, CT) 结合系统。利用这套系统，为患者做 CT 和 PET 成像过程中，没必要改变他们的体位；同时也可以获得集功能、解剖于一体的影像。另外，CT 扫描同样是对人体的透射扫描，可以利用 CT 扫描来校正光电子在患者体内的衰减。它还有另外的优点，就是利用 CT 扫描来为衰减影像采集必要的信息时，在很大程度上可减少检查时间。

 答案

Positron emission tomography (PET) is now routinely used for clinical imaging. Results of previous studies have shown that the detection of lesions deep in the body with PET is improved with correction for the attenuation of photons. Recently, PET/computed tomography (CT) combined system has been introduced by different manufacturers. With such system it is possible to image patients with PET and CT without the need to change their position. Besides, it can obtain co-registered functional-anatomic images. In addition, the CT scan is also a transmission scan of the body, and therefore it is possible to use the CT scan to correct for the attenuation of photons within the patient. Making use of a CT scan to acquire the necessary information for an attenuation map has the added advantage of considerably reducing the examination time.

Positron emission tomography 正电子发射断层显像技术，简称 PET
attenuation [ətenju'eiʃən] *n.* 衰减　　photon ['fəutɔn] *n.* 光子
manufacturer [ˌmænju'fæktʃərə] *n.* 厂商
functional ['fʌŋkʃənl] *a.* 功能的、函数的
transmission [trænz'miʃən] *n.* 透射、发射、传输
to the advantage of 对……有利

第 50 天

 学习

Stereotaxic technique is used in neurosurgery for intracranial biopsies and in radiation

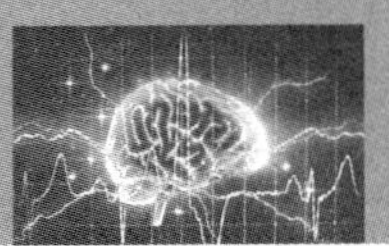

therapy for focal irradiation of intracranial targets. The target localization procedures use stereotaxic frames and modern imaging techniques such as CT, MR imaging, and digital subtraction angiography (DSA). A reference marker box is fitted to the stereotaxic frame during the imaging sessions, producing reference markers in the image. Coordinates of specific points of interest within the brain are determined in the stereotaxic frame coordinate system by using these reference markers. Separate marker boxes are used for imaging with CT, MR, and DSA, because each imaging technique requires either a unique material to produce the marker in the image (CT and MR) or a unique geometry (DSA). Both MR imaging and CT may be needed to assess a particular intracranial lesion, necessitating changing the marker box on the patient when moving from the MR to the CT scanner. Determining an inexpensive substance for contrast material for CT and MR, especially one that is available in radiology departments, would help with acquiring images for radiosurgery treatments. Therefore, we have tested various contrast materials normally found in radiology departments to find a material that could be used with both CT and MR imaging without causing significant artifacts or distortion on either type of image.

立体定向技术用于神经外科颅内病变的活检和放疗中颅内靶点的灶性照射。使用立体定向仪和现代影像技术，诸如 CT、MRI 和数字减影血管造影（digital subtraction angiography，DSA）确定靶点位置。在成像断层时，此参考标记箱适合于立体定向仪，可在影像上产生参考标记。用这些参考标记在立体定向仪坐标系中确定颅内兴趣区的坐标。由于各种成像技术要求用一种物质在影像内产生标记（CT 和 MR）或几何图形（DSA），个别的标记箱用于 CT、MR 和 DSA 成像。MRI 和 CT 都要对颅内病变做出诊断，当患者从 MR 移动到 CT 扫描时就须改变标记箱。确定一种用于 CT 和 MR 价廉的对比剂，尤其是放射科常用的，能帮助放射外科治疗获得影像。因此我们测试了放射科内易得到的各种对比剂，以便发现一种既能用于 CT，又能用于 MRI，且在每幅图像上都不产生伪影或失真的物质。

neurosurgery ['njuərəusə:dʒəri] *n.* 神经外科学

intracranial [ˌintrə'kreiniəl] *a.* 颅内的

biopsy ['baiɔpsi] *vt.* 活检

radiation therapy 放射治疗

frame [freim] *n.* 框架

digital subtraction angiography 数字减影血管造影

coordinate [kəu'ɔ:dinit] *n.* 坐标系

distortion [di'stɔ:ʃn] *n.* 变形、失真

focal ['fəukəl] *a.* 焦点的

irradiation [ireidi'eiʃən] *n.* 照射、辐射

localization [ˌləukəlai'zeiʃn] *n.* 定位、局限

selective localization 选择性定位

particular [pə'tikjulə] *a.* 特别的；in particular 特别是、尤其是

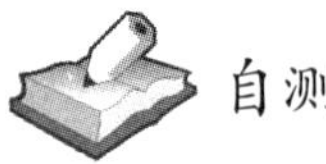
自测

在磁共振成像（magnetic resonance imaging，MRI）检查中，颅脑的轴位影像已被列入常规，但因在轴位影像成角度数方面没有统一的标准，故要比较轴位 MRI 检查与后来的 MRI 检查或与计算机断层扫描（computed tomographic，CT) 检查相比较就很困难。

答案

Axial images of the brain are routinely acquired during magnetic resonance (MR) imaging examination. However, there is no standard for the degree of angulation in axial images. This lack of a standard makes it difficult to compare axial MR imaging examination with subsequent MR imaging examination or computed tomographic (CT) examination.

magnetic resonance imaging 磁共振成像，简称 MRI

angulation [ˌæŋgju'leiʃən] *n.* 角度

第 51 天

学习

For CT of the brain, there are three standard reference lines: the orbitomeatal line, the Reid baseline, and the supraorbitomeatal line. The orbitomeatal line runs through the external canthus and the center of the external auditory meatus. This is the most widely used line, because acquisition of fewer sections is necessary to cover the entire brain. The Reid baseline runs though the inferior orbital wall and the superior border of the external auditory meatus. This line is parallel to the optic nerve and provides the best demonstration of the orbital contents. The supraorbitomeatal line runs through the superior orbital wall and the center of the external auditory meatus. This line approximately parallels the skull base.We developed reference lines for use at MR imaging that are analogous to the three standard reference lines used at CT, on the basis of anatomic landmarks that are visible on midsagittal MR images.These lines can be used to prescribe subsequent oblique axial sequences.

对于颅脑 CT 有三个标准参考线：听眦线、里德基线和眶上线。听眦线通过外眦至外耳道中心，被广为使用，因为用它来覆盖全部颅脑时所用切面较少。里德基线经过眶下壁至外耳道的上缘，平行于视神经并提供眶内容物的最佳显示。眶上线经过眶上壁至外耳道中心，与颅底大约平行。基于正中矢状面 MR 影像上可视的解剖标志，我们创立了与 CT 的三条标准参考线相似的用于 MR 成像的参考线。这些参考线可以用于指定倾斜轴位的序列。

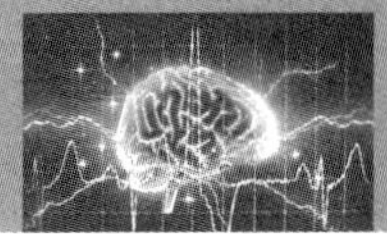

orbitomeatal line 听眦线
orbit ['ɔ:bit] *n.* 眶，轨道
anatomic landmark 解剖标志
Reid baseline 里德基线（连接眶下嵴至外耳道及枕区中线之线，用于测颅）
supraorbitomeatal line 眶上线
external [ik'stə:nl] *a.* 外的、外部的
canthus ['kænθəs] *n.* 眦，眼角；复数 canthi ['kænθai]
auditory ['ɔ:ditəri] *a.* 听的、听觉的
meatus [mi'eitəs] *n.* 道；复数 meatus（es）
inferior [in'fiəriə] *a.* 下方的
optic ['ɔptik] *a.* 眼的
skull [skʌl] *n.* 头颅骨
sagittal ['sædʒətəl] *a.* 矢状的
subsequent ['sʌbsikwənt] *a.* 随后的
oblique [ə'bli:k] *a.* 斜的
sequence ['si:kwəns] *n.* 连续、顺序、定序

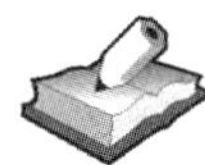

自测

通过乳腺 X 线摄影普查来降低死亡率需要高质量的检查。检查的技术和临床方面的因素都会影响乳腺 X 线照片质量。技术质量评价包括用标准测试物（体模）对成像设备的评价，以确认适合所用胶片的洗片机的评价，以及对乳腺施行放射剂量的测定。临床影像质量评价包括对某种设备所产生的胶片的评价和对摄影位置、乳腺压迫、对比度、曝光、噪声、锐利度、伪影及标记的考虑。

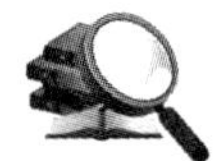

答案

Achieving mortality reduction through screening mammography requires high-quality examination. Both technical and clinical aspects of the examination affect mammographic quality. Technical quality assessment includes evaluation of imaging equipment with a standardized test object (phantom), evaluation of the processor to be sure it is appropriately set for the used film, and measurement of the radiation dose to the breast. Clinical image quality assessment involves review of the films produced by a facility and consideration of positioning, breast compression, contrast, exposure, noise, sharpness, artifacts, and labeling.

mortality [mɔ:'tæliti] *n.* 致命性、死亡率
processor ['prəusesə] *n.* 洗片机
radiation dose 放射剂量
facility [fə'siliti] *n.* 容易、可能性

第 52 天

学习

Screening mammography is the most effective means of early detection of breast cancer. However, a screening program can be successful, only if eligible women actually undergo the procedure. Though utilization rates have been increasing over the past several years, the initiative goal of 60% screening of more than 50 year-old women, as set forth in the Healthy People 2000 by the United States Department of Health and Human Services, has not yet been achieved. Numerous published studies have revealed a variety of barriers between physicians and patients that prevent women from undergoing screening. Two commonly cited barriers are cost and convenience. Many innovative strategies have been devised in an attempt to overcome some of these barriers.

进行乳腺X线照相普查是诊断早期乳腺癌最有效的方法。然而，只有当符合条件的妇女确实进行了这项检查，此项普查计划才算成功。尽管过去多年普查率逐渐上升，但2000年美国卫生与人文服务部的“健康人群”计划中提出的60%的50岁以上的妇女进行普查的目标，还是没能实现。许多发表的研究揭示医患之间的各种障碍阻止了妇女接受普查。成本和便利性是两个常涉及的障碍。因此，已经设计了许多试图克服这些障碍的创新方法。

eligible ['elidʒəbl] *a.* 符合被推选条件的　　devise [di'vaiz] *v.* 设计、创造、产生
strategy ['strætidʒi] *n.* 战略、对策　　physician [fi'ziʃən] *n.* 医师

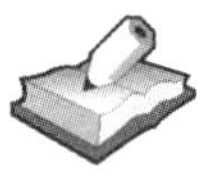

自测

放射界十分注重乳腺X线摄影的质量控制，并考虑到许多细节如X线洗片机、屏-片组合、乳腺X线摄影发生器和X线管。可是，对乳腺X线观片灯及其观片条件考虑得太少。

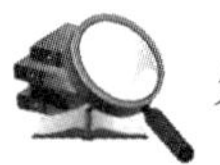

答案

The radiology community has focused much attention on quality control in mammography, considering such details as the photographic processor, the film-screen combination, and the mammographic generator and X-ray tube. However, little consideration has been given to the mammographic viewboxes and viewing conditions.

quality control 质量控制，简称QC　　film-screen combination 屏-片组合

第53天

学习

Some data are available regarding the effects of viewing conditions on the detection of low-contrast image details. Extraneous light has been shown to decrease the detectability of low-contrast details. However, seeing adjacent viewboxes left on while no films are on them is still common. Furthermore, low viewbox luminance levels reduce the ability to detect small details, especially at high film optical densities.

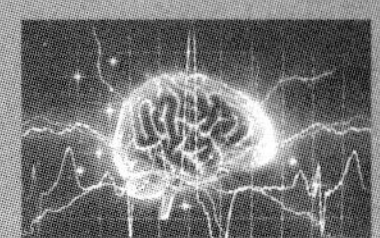

有一些关于观片条件在低对比影像细节诊断上作用的数据表明，额外光线可降低低对比细节的检出率。可是，相邻观片灯开着而没有照片的情况屡见不鲜。此外，观片灯低亮度可降低对小细节的诊断，尤其在照片高光学密度时更是这样。

extraneous[ek'streiniəs]*a.* 外部的　　luminance level 亮度

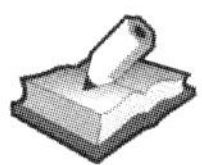

自测

今后 10 年在许多医学中心，直接获取的数字乳腺 X 线摄影将可能取代屏 - 片乳腺 X 线摄影。尽管我们学院放射科的其他领域都已成功地过渡到数字影像，但乳腺 X 线摄影还没能数字化。转变成数字影像的一个最大障碍是微小钙化和肿块边缘的探测和特性描述对高分辨率的需求。

答案

Direct-acquisition digital mammography is likely to supplant screen-film mammography at many medical centers over the next decade. Despite the successful transition to digital imaging of all other areas of radiology in our institution, mammography has not yet become digital. A major impediment to conversion to digital imaging is the demanding for high resolution required for detection and characterization of microcalcifications and the margins of mass.

supplant[sə'plɑ:nt]*vt.* 取代

impediment[im'pedimənt]*n.* 阻碍、障碍；a major impediment to　……的主要障碍

margin['mɑ:dʒin]*n.* 边缘　　mass[mæs]*n.* 肿块

screen-film mammography 屏 - 片乳腺 X 线摄影

第 54 天

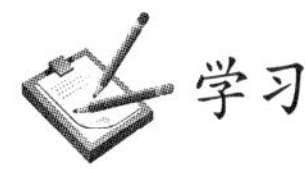

学习

One of the most novel and promising methods for meeting the technical challenge of full-field direct digital mammography is slot scanning. This technique uses a narrow X-ray beam that sweeps across the object to be imaged synchronously with a narrow array of charge coupled devices on a detector below the object. As the photons pass through the object, proportional electronic signals are transmitted from the detector, first to an analog-to-digital converter and then to a computer that creates the image for display. A unique advantage of this system over others proposed for digital mammography is substantially reduced image degradation from scatter radiation. Shared with other direct digital mammography systems is the advantage over screen-film mammography of separating image acquisition, display, and storage so that each can be optimized.

为应对全视野直接数字乳腺X线摄影所遇到的技术挑战，最新且有前途的方法之一便是裂隙扫描。此项技术采用狭窄的X线束扫描物体，而物体下探测器具有一组狭窄的电荷耦合器同步移动成像。当光子通过物体时，从探测器发出相应的电子信号，首先到模数转换器，然后再到计算机产生图像显示。对于数字乳腺X线摄影此系统较其他方法独特的优势是显著地减少了来自散射线的影像降级。和其他直接数字乳腺X线摄影系统一样，相对于屏-片乳腺X线摄影，其优势是把影像获取、显示和存储分开，使得每项都能最优化。

novel ['nɔvl] *a.* 新颖的

full-field direct digital mammography 全视野直接数字乳腺X线摄影

sweep [swi:p](swept, swept) *v.* 扫描

synchronously ['siŋkrənəsli] *ad.* 同时发生地、同步地

analog-to-digital converter 模数转换器，简称ADC　　scatter radiation 散射线

substantial [səb'stænʃəl] *a.* 物质的、实际的、坚固的、重要的

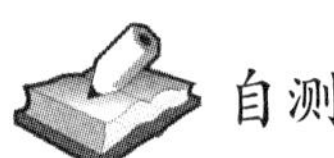

自测

此系统主要的关注焦点之一是其获取影像需要相对较长的时间——6.9 s，是许多患者采用屏-片技术曝光时间的3倍还要多。在获得影像时，较长时间的曝光增加了患者移动所致伪影的风险，且增加了人们对显示癌症细微征象，如聚集的微钙化结果模糊的担忧。

答案

One of the chief concerns about this system is its relatively long image acquisition time, 6.9 sec, which is more than three times the exposure time used for most patients with the screen-film technique. A longer exposure increases the risk of artifact from patient motion during image acquisition and has raised concern about resultant obscuration of subtle signs of cancer such as clustered microcalcifications.

resultant [ri'zʌltənt] *n.* 结果　　obscuration [ɔbskjuə'reiʃən] *n.* 模糊

cluster ['klʌstə] *v.* 成群、群集、簇集

第55天

学习

Digital mammography is considered to be the technique that has “the greatest potential impact on the management of breast cancer”. In digital mammography, image acquisition, storage and display are performed independently, allowing optimization of each stage. Unlike conventional imaging, which requires low X-ray energy to ensure high contrast of the film, digital

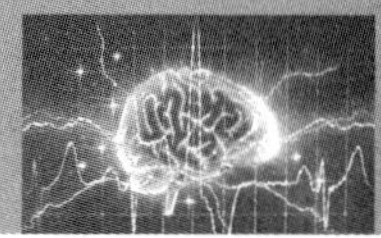

detector permits wider variation in the X-ray energy.

数字乳腺 X 线摄影被认为是“在乳腺癌监控方面最具潜力”的技术。在数字乳腺 X 线摄影中，影像获取、存储及显示是独立完成的，且使每步最优化。与传统成像需要窄 X 线能级以确保胶片的高对比不一样，数字探测器允许较宽的各种 X 线能级。

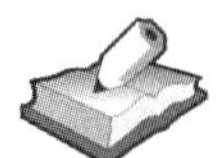

自测

传统乳腺 X 线摄影的空间分辨率高达 20 lp/mm。为达到这个指标，数字乳腺 X 线摄影在小区域数字探测器中像素大小远比不上当前达到的 0.025 mm。空间分辨率是传统乳腺 X 线摄影的强项之一。但是有一些资料显示，由于对比细节的改善，分辨率少于 10 lp/mm 的数字乳腺 X 线摄影比屏 - 片乳腺 X 线摄影有更好的病变诊断能力。因此，研究比较屏 - 片乳腺 X 线摄影与高空间分辨率的数字乳腺 X 线摄影是很有必要的。先前的调查研究已比较了数字化屏 - 片乳腺 X 线摄影，但数字影像的质量受胶片上原始信息质量的限制。在数字处理中信息也可能丢失。这些研究表明在数字化胶片与模拟影像间在病灶的诊断方面无显著性差异。

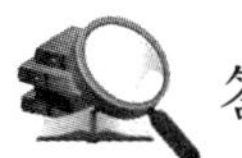

答案

The spatial resolution of conventional mammography is up to 20 line pairs per millimetre (lp/mm). To achieve this, digital mammography must have pixels spaced no further apart than 0.025 mm which is currently achievable only in small field digital detector. Spatial resolution is one of the strengths of conventional mammography. However, there is some evidence suggesting that digital mammography with a resolution less than 10 lp/mm may have better lesion detectability than screen–film mammography owing to the improved contrast detail. Therefore, research comparing screen–film mammography and digital mammography with high spatial resolution is much needed. Previous research studies have used digitized screen–film mammography for comparison, but the quality of the digital image remained limited by the quality of the original information on the film. During the digitization process, there was also a possibility of information loss. These studies reported no significant difference in lesion detection between the digitized film and analog image.

line pairs per millimetre 每毫米线对（lp/mm）

第 56 天

学习

Some studies compared storage phosphors with conventional screen–film mammography. It was found that computed radiography approached the performance of screen–film mammography for survey views, but may be superior to screen–film mammography in the detection of microcalcifications in a spot view. However, studies comparing charge coupled device (CCD) imaging detector for digital mammography and conventional mammography are limited. One such study found that the contrast detail detectability of the digital system was significantly superior to the conventional system.

一些研究比较了存储荧光与传统屏 - 片乳腺 X 线摄影。调查发现计算机 X 线摄影（computed radiography, CR）接近屏 - 片乳腺 X 线摄影的性能，但在微小钙化的诊断方面可能优于屏 - 片乳腺 X 线摄影。但是对电子耦合器件（charge coupled device, CCD）成像探测器的数字乳腺 X 线摄影与传统乳腺 X 线摄影的对比研究还很少。一项此类研究发现数字系统的对比细节诊断率明显优于传统系统。

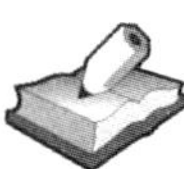 自测

临床上尽可能早期检查到小的乳腺癌，对降低其死亡率是很有价值的。在无症状的妇女身上检测隐匿性乳腺癌是乳腺 X 线摄影的主要功能。然而，遗憾的是，尽管乳腺 X 线摄影对乳腺癌的发现十分敏感，但乳腺 X 线摄影仅能见到形态学的变化，对乳腺良、恶性肿瘤的鉴别常显不足。经常必须定位穿刺活检确定乳腺 X 线摄影所见病变的原因。

 答案

Detection of a breast cancer lesion at a smaller size and earlier stage that is possible at clinical examination has been shown to be efficacious in reducing mortality from breast cancer. The detection of clinically occult breast cancer in an asymptomatic woman is the principal function of mammography. Unfortunately, although mammography is quite sensitive for the detection of breast cancer, morphologic criteria that are mammographically visible are frequently insufficient for the differentiation of benign from malignant lesions. Performance of needle aspiration and needle localization procedures followed by excisional biopsy is frequently necessary to determine the origin of a mammographic finding.

efficacious [efi'keiʃəs] *a.* 有效的　　benign [bi'nain] *a.* 良性的
asymptomatic [ˌeisimptə'mætik] *a.* 无症状的
morphologic [ˌmɔːfə'lɔdʒik] *n.* 形态学　　malignant [mə'lignənt] *a.* 恶性的
excision [ek'siʒən] *n.* 切除　　aspiration [ˌæspə'reiʃən] *n.* 吸引术、抽吸

第 57 天

 学习

The direction of needle insertion must reproduce the path taken by the X-ray beam on the

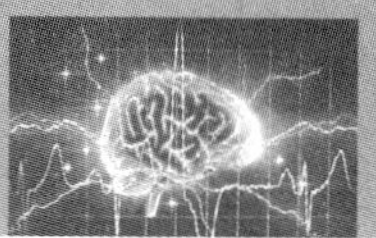

preliminary radiograph as it traversed the tissues. Since the X-ray beam is divergent, this path is frequently not perpendicular to the film surface, and if accuracy is to be achieved the operator must angle the needle to parallel the path of the incident X-ray beam. This is accomplished with use of the field light or laser that is mounted in the X-ray collimator and various crosshair devices to define the point at which the X-ray beam passed through the skin on its path through the lesion. The tip of the needle is placed at this point.

当穿刺针通过组织时，其进入的方向必须与预照片 X 线通过的方向一致。由于 X 线是扩散的，其径路常常不垂直于胶片表面，如果要达到准确定位，必须使穿刺针平行于入射的 X 线束。这就需要使用缩光器或激光来完成，即在 X 线机上安装准直器和不同的十字基准线附件，以确定 X 线束通过皮肤及其径路到达病变，针尖就置于该点。

divergent [dai'vəːdʒənt] *a.* 发散的、辐射状的　　angle ['æŋgl] *n.* 角度

perpendicular [pəːpən'dikjulə] *a.* 与……垂直的（to）　　laser ['leizə] *n.* 激光

incident ['insidənt] *a.* 入射的　　mount [maunt] *v.* 安装

mount M in N 把 M 镶嵌在 N 里；mount M on N 把 M 安装在 N 上；mount up 安装

collimator ['kɔlimeitə] *n.* 准直器

crosshair ['krɔːshɛə] *n.* 十字准线　　skin [skin] *n.* 皮肤

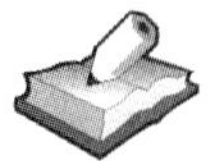

自测

随着磁共振成像（magnetic resonance imaging, MRI）乳腺检诊的进步，被 MRI 检出的乳腺可疑病变的患者也随之增加。目前，就本组病例而言，手术切除病变或短期内 MR 复查是一个重要的诊断手段。近来，我们采取在 MR 原配的活检线圈上加上一个立体引导装置，即改变一下主机的表面线圈用作活检线圈，这种简单安全而又用途广泛的装置，有利于 MR 准确引导细针活检。

答案

As the frequency of magnetic resonance (MR) imaging examinations of the breast increases, so does the number of suspect lesions detected exclusively with this imaging modality. At present, performance of surgical excision of the approximate region or short-term MR follow-up is the only diagnostic option in such cases. Prototypes of biopsy coils have been presented recently. We have developed an add-on guiding device that transforms a commercially available surface coil into a biopsy coil. This simple and versatile unit permits performance of accurate MR-guided needle biopsies.

surface coil 表面线圈　　versatile ['vəːsətail] *a.* 通用的、万能的

modality [məu'dæləti] *n.* 模态、方式

第 58 天

学习

Contrast enhancement pattern is one of the most important diagnostic clues for evaluation of lesions at magnetic resonance (MR) imaging in the breast. Depending on the sequence parameters, it may be impossible to differentiate between small islands of fat and enhancing lesions without performing time-consuming comparison of the precontrast and postcontrast images. Two different approaches to attain more conspicuity of lesion enhancement are available: the fat-suppression technique and the subtraction technique. Inhomogeneity of signal intensity and increased measurement time are relevant disadvantages of the fat-suppression technique. For this reason, the subtraction technique is popular with many investigators. However, this technique has a well-known vulnerability of motion artifacts. Motion of the patient during measurement creates both low-intensity and high-intensity bands of signal extinction, which diminishes the image quality. A simple compression device was therefore developed to reduce motion artifacts on routinely obtained diagnostic breast MR images with commercially available breast surface coils.

在乳腺磁共振（magnetic resonance，MR）成像中，对比增强形态对于评价病变是最重要的诊断思路之一。依据序列参数，如果不做耗费时间的增强前后图像对比就可能无法鉴别小的脂肪岛和增强病变。有两种不同的方法能够实现病变增强的显著性：脂肪抑制技术和减影技术。脂肪抑制技术中信号强度不均和测量时间的增加是两个相关弱点。正因如此，减影技术被许多研究者们普遍采用。但这技术有一个众所周知的弱点——移动伪影。在检查期间患者移动产生信号消失的低强度和高强度带，降低了影像质量。为此，我们开发了一个简单的压迫装置，以便在常规乳腺线圈 MR 成像中减少移动伪影。

parameter［pə'ræmitə］*n.* 参数　　conspicuity *n.* 能见度

inhomogeneity［'in,həuməd3i'ni:iti］*n.* 不均匀性

suppression［sə'preʃən］*n.* 抑制　　fat-suppression technique 脂肪抑制技术

subtraction［səb'trækʃən］*n.* 减去　　vulnerability［vʌlnərə'biliti］*n.* 弱点

extinction *n.* 衰减　　diminish［di'miniʃ］*v.* 减少、缩小、递减、削弱

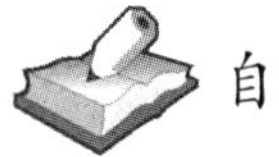

自测

虽然自 1929 年起就能通过电话传输 X 线照片，但更先进的系统一直在缓慢引进。我们描述一个简便的系统，通过个人的计算机和因特万维网系统传递医学影像。

答案

Although the ability to transmit radiographs over the telephone has been feasible since 1929,

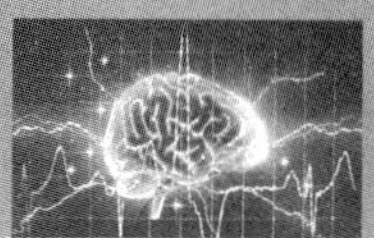

more advanced systems have been in slow introduction. We describe a simple system for transmitting medical images across a system based on personal computers and the internet's world wide web.

第 59 天

学习

Most hospitals in the United States have fewer than 100 beds. Different studies have shown that 20%—59% of radiology practices have fewer than five radiologists. As many as 26% of practices consist of one or two radiologists. In small and often rural hospitals, the volume of radiologic studies cannot justify having an in-house radiologist throughout the night.

在美国大多数医院少于 100 张床位。各种研究显示 20% ~ 59% 的放射科拥有少于 5 位的放射学家。26% 的放射科也只有 1 位或 2 位放射学家。在小医院，尤其是郊区医院，也不能保证一整夜由 1 名放射医生值班来完成放射检查。

radiologist *n.* 放射学家　　rural ['ruərəl] *a.* 农村的

justify ['dʒʌstifai] *vt.* 证明为正当，为……辩护

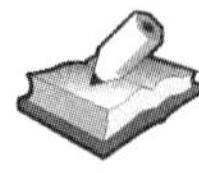
自测

一些研究已经报道了从激光 - 数字化传统 X 线照片能做出准确诊断。许多远程放射学系统的费用是非常昂贵的，尤其对于小医院的大量急诊检查。在我们 55 张床的郊外社区医院，我们希望 1 位放射学家对所有急诊核医学、超声图像及 CT 研究能立即提供初步的判读。

答案

Several studies have reported accurate diagnosis from laser-digitized conventional radiographs. The costs of many teleradiology systems can be prohibitive, especially for the volume of emergent studies in small hospitals. At our 55-bed rural community hospital we prefer that a radiologist provide an immediate preliminary interpretation of all emergency nuclear medicine, sonographic, can and CT studies.

emergency [i'mə:dʒənsi] *n.* 急症

emergent [i'mə:dʒənt] *a.* 紧急的、意外的

nuclear ['nju:kliə] *a.* (原子)核的　　medicine ['medisin] *n.* 医学

sonographic [ˌsəunəu'græfik] *a.* 超声检查的

prohibitive [prə'hibitiv] *a.* 禁止的、抑制的　　community hospital 社区医院

第 60 天

学习

With the rapid development of PACS in radiology, digital image interpretation is being introduced at an ever-growing number of hospitals. The technical, financial, and practical advantages of digital radiology can be exploited to their full potential only when image evaluation relies solely on soft-copy display. Results of several previous studies in various areas of diagnostic imaging have shown that soft-copy image quality is at least comparable to conventional hard-copy imaging and that primary soft-copy evaluation is feasible. Most of these studies used cathode ray tube (CRT) displays and focused on the impact of technical parameters, such as luminescence, spatial resolution or data processing, and diagnostic performance.

随着放射学 PACS 的快速发展,数目众多的医院引进了数字影像判读。当影像评价唯一依赖于软拷贝显示时,数字放射学才能充分发挥其潜在的技术、资金和实际优势。先前在成像诊断领域进行的一些研究结果表明软拷贝影像质量至少可以与传统硬拷贝成像质量相比,软拷贝初步评价是可行的。这些研究绝大部分采用阴极射线管(cathode ray tube, CRT)显示,重点研究技术参数的影响,如发光、空间分辨率、数据处理和诊断性能。

soft-copy display 软拷贝显示　　feasible ['fi:zəbl] *a.* 可行的

conventional hard-copy imaging 传统硬拷贝成像

cathode ray tube 阴极射线管,简称 CRT

financial [fai'nænʃəl] *a.* 财政上的,财务的

exploit [iks'plɔit] *vt.* 开发、利用　　solely ad. 独自、完全

solely responsible 单独负责的　　solely because of 只是因为……缘故

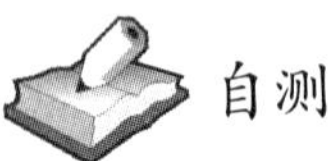

自测

电子用户通常使用液晶显示 (liquid crystal displays, LCD),但近来已被引入到放射学的软拷贝判读上。与 CRT 相比,LCD 显示的特点是较小矩阵尺寸、较高的低对比分辨率和较大的动态范围。尽管初步研究描述了每块板相对高的像素丢失(“黑洞”),但现在大多数文章报道了其优越的空间分辨率、良好的均一性和模糊炫光几乎完全消除。用 LCD 进行诊断评价实验很有限。一项对键盘使用、显示器的可接受性及显示尺寸方面的评价问卷调查并没发现 LCD 与 CRT 显示有显著性差异。据我们所知,临床上诊断性能、更多的影像质量特性评价未能在更深层次上涉及。

答案

Liquid crystal displays (LCD) are common in consumer electronics but only recently

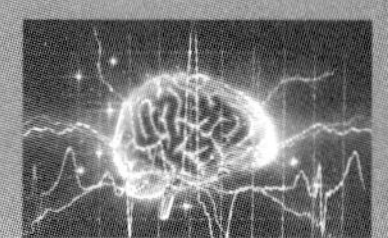

have been introduced for soft-copy interpretations in radiology. Compared with CRT displays, LCD are characterized by a smaller matrix size but a higher small-spot contrast ratio and larger dynamic range. Although initial studies described a relatively high number of missing pixels ("black holes") per panel, most recent publications reported excellent spatial resolution and a high uniformity and almost complete elimination of veiling glare. Experience with LCD for diagnostic evaluation is limited. A questionnaire that evaluated keyboard usage, acceptability of monitor screen, and display size did not find significant differences between the LCD and the CRT displays. No further evaluations of diagnostic performance or more specific assessments of image quality in a clinical setting have been performed, to our knowledge.

liquid crystal displays 液晶显示，简称 LCD

larger dynamic range 较大的动态范围

matrix size 矩阵大小　　　veil [veil] *n.* 模糊、遮蔽物

第 61 天

学习

During the past decade, many investigators have addressed the feasibility of picture archiving and communication system (PACS) as an alternative to film-based radiology. To successfully implement the PACS, a number of factors such as film resolution, interpretation conditions, and a cost-effective viewer system must be taken into consideration. The most important clinical criterion for using the PACS technology is the ability to achieve acceptable accuracy when interpreting radiologic images at a soft-copy viewing workstation. Most previous reports have focused on a comparison of observer performance with soft-copy and hard-copy images, and such studies have been performed using chest radiography. However, observer performance in projection radiography of another anatomic section must also be compared to achieve that the PACS can completely replace film-based radiology.

过去 10 年里，许多研究者已经提出了图像存储与传输系统（picture archiving and communication systems, PACS）替代胶片放射学的可行性。为成功实现 PACS，必须考虑胶片分辨率、判读环境及成本 - 效益检查系统等因素。使用 PACS 技术最重要的一项临床标准是当在软拷贝观察工作站判读 X 线影像时图片显示能够达到可接受的正确性。许多研究者先前的报告集中比较软拷贝与硬拷贝影像的性能，且这些研究是采用胸部 X 线摄影来进行的。但观察者必须比较其他解剖部位的 X 线照片的性能，以期实现 PACS 完全取代以胶片为基础的放射学。

picture archiving and communication systems 图像存档与传输系统，简称 PACS

at a soft-copy viewing workstation 软拷贝观察工作站

implement ['implimənt] *v.* 实现、完成

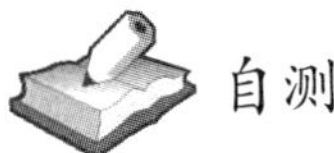

自测

最近一项报告显示，传统观片灯与大多数软拷贝相比在显示的亮度方面存在大的差异。因为缺乏能产生较亮影像而保持分辨率及对比灵敏度的成本 - 效益软拷贝观察技术，已经花费了许多努力试图明确亮度的不均匀性。如果想在 PACS 临床上成功，必须考虑亮度特性以及分辨率性能。到目前为止，高分辨率 2K × 2K 的影像显示器已做为 PACS 软拷贝显示系统而被广泛运用。但在无胶片成像的环境中，要在临床实践中广泛地应用这种昂贵的显示器可能不符合成本 - 效益管理。因此，我们必须考虑一种能替代高分辨率影像显示器，符合成本 - 效益管理的机器，这种机器可以得到同样有效的图像。

答案

A recent report showed that large differences in luminance exist between conventional viewbox displays and most soft-copy displays. Because of a lack of cost-effective soft-copy viewing technology that yields brighter images while preserving resolution and contrast sensitivity, much effort has been expended in an attempt to define nonuniformities in luminance. If PACS is to succeed in the clinical environment, both the luminance factor and the resolution factor must be taken into account. Until now, high-resolution video monitor of 2K × 2K has been widely used as a soft-copy viewing system for PACS. However, in the environment of filmless imaging, the universal use of this expensive monitor in clinical practice may not be cost-effective. Therefore, we must consider an alternative to the high-resolution video monitor that is cost-effective and that can present images as effectively as the high-resolution monitor.

第 62 天

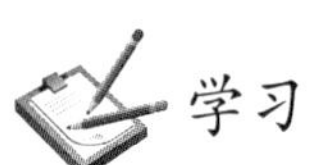

学习

PACS has changed the workflow of radiology department and the radiologist's way to evaluate radiologic examinations. Cross-sectional imaging methods, including MRI, are best suited to handling a PACS workstation, because data are directly available in digital format, and the software tools available on the PACS workstation may facilitate evaluations of large numbers of images compared with the classic viewing of hard copies on viewboxes, and because the requirements with regard to computer screens are not as stringent as for chest radiography or mammography. Several studies have evaluated the effect of PACS on radiologists' productivity and accuracy for thoracoabdominal CT, mammography, conventional chest radiography, and conventional skeletal radiography. To date, little has been published on PACS-based image

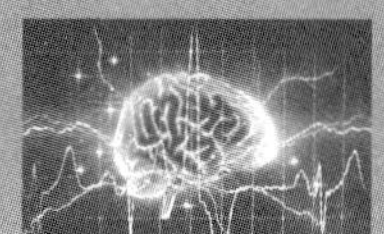

interpretation of MR images, especially in the field of musculoskeletal MRI.

PACS 已经改变放射科的工作流程和放射学家对放射检查的评价方式。断面成像方法，包括 MRI，是最适合于 PACS 工作站处理，因为可以直接获得数字格式的数据，且 PACS 工作站里用的软件工具使得大量的图像比在硬拷贝观片灯上评价更便利，还因为电脑屏幕的要求不像胸部 X 线照片或乳腺 X 线照片那样严格。一些研究已经评估了放射学家采用 PACS 对胸腹 CT、乳腺 X 线摄影、常规胸部 X 线摄影以及常规骨骼 X 线摄影检查效率和准确性所产生的作用。到目前为止，几乎还没有发表有关以 PACS 为基础的 MR 图像的判读，特别是在骨骼肌 MRI 领域。

skeletal ['skelətl] *a.* 骨骼的　　thoracoabdominal [ˌθɔːrəkəuəb'dɔminl] *a.* 胸腹的

musculoskeletal [ˌmʌskjuləu'skelətəl] *a.* 肌与骨骼的

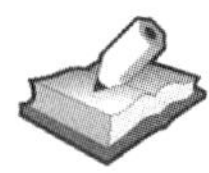

自测

放射学家们长期以来因为缺乏一种可提取和存储感兴趣影像的简单系统而受到困扰。单纯采用观片灯、三脚架、相机和暗室去收集各种不同疾病的影像范例导致大量的影像丢失。拷贝胶片制作费用昂贵，体积庞大难以管理和存储，笨重难以携带。图像存储和传输系统（picture archiving and communication system, PACS）的出现大大提高了图像显示的速度及其灵活性。然而，大多数 PACS 系统没能提供为临床 PACS 环境以外提取使用影像的有效方法而令许多放射学家失望。PACS 执照的发行往往阻碍了放射科试图把影像提取软件装到所有人 PACS 系统的原代码中。结果，许多放射学家必须承担分离、费时的步骤去提取医学数字成像与传输（digital imaging and communications in medicine, DICOM），或从他们的 PACS 中提取其他所有人的影像，把它们下载到可移动的媒介，然后将这些影像转换成更便于使用的格式。

答案

Radiologists have long been plagued by the lack of a simple system of capturing and storing interesting images. The tedium of using viewboxes, tripods, cameras, and darkrooms to collect images illustrating good examples of various diseases has been responsible for the loss of many such images. Copied films are expensive to create, bulky to organize and store, and heavy to move. The advent of picture archiving and communication system (PACS) has brought tremendous speed and flexibility to film display. Unfortunately, many radiologists have been disappointed to find that most PACS systems fail to offer an efficient means of capturing images for use outside the clinical PACS environment. PACS licensing issue generally prevents radiology department from attempting to incorporate image-capture software into the proprietary primary code of their PACS system. As a result, many radiologists must undertake separate, time-consuming steps to capture digital imaging and communications in medicine (DICOM) or other proprietary images from their PACS, download them to a removable medium, and then convert these images to more usable formats.

plague [pleig] *vt.* 烦扰、使苦恼

tedium ['ti:diəm] *n.* 单调、冗长乏味、沉闷

tripod ['traipɔd] *n.* 三脚架

illustrate ['iləstreit] *v.* 图解、举例说明

bulky ['bʌlki] *a.* 体积大的、笨重的

tremendous [trə'mendəs] *a.* 可怕的、惊人的

flexibility [ˌfleksə'biliti] *n.* 灵活性、机动性

incorporate [in'kɔ:pəreit] *v.* 插入；incorporate M in (into) N 把 M 引入 N

proprietary [prə'praiətəri] *a.* 所有人的、专有的

digital imaging and communications in medicine 医学数字成像与传输，简称 DICOM

第 63 天

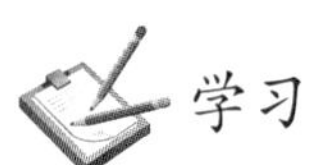
学习

We have implemented a system that operates on our departmental PCs and PACS workstations and allows the efficient capture and transfer of images from the PACS system to a stand-alone server. Users capture images “on the fly” from PACS workstations, without interrupting workflow, and the system saves the images to a server. The user can later annotate, file, organize, store, retrieve, and display the images without tying up PACS resources. Our system renders the issue of ensuring unnecessary compatibility with DICOM because we based our system on screen capturing rather than on the direct pulling of DICOM images from a PACS server.

我们实行一种可在我们科室个人电脑和 PACS 工作站运行的系统，从 PACS 系统可有效提取和传递图像到可独立应用的服务器中。在没有干扰工作流程的情况下，用户从 PACS 工作站中“飞似的”提取影像，此系统将影像储存到服务器。之后用户不占用 PACS 资源就可以注释、归档、管理、存储、检索和显示影像。因为我们的系统是基于屏幕提取影像，而不是从一个 PACS 服务器中直接提取 DICOM 影像，因此，我们的系统提供确保无需与 DICOM 兼容的版本。

annotate ['ænəteit] *v.* 注释、注解

retrieve [ri'tri:v] *vt.* 重新得到、取回

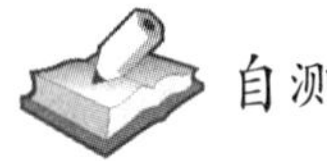
自测

我们的系统由于从 PACS 环境中转移拷贝影像，并立即将它们转到另一个服务器中，因而消除了工作流程冲突。通过从 PACS 服务器中分离非临床影像服务器，我们保护了 PACS 的临床性能。让 PACS 工作站的利用率最大化，而在 PACS 网上的通讯减至最小。因为网上

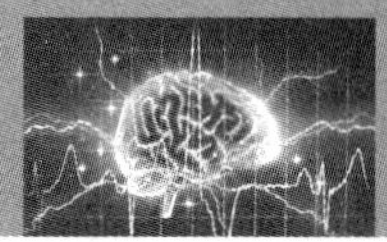

的任何计算机（不仅仅是 PACS 工作站）能被用于操作和显示拷贝影像，所以我们的系统增加了获取影像的方法。

答案

Our system eliminates workflow conflicts by removing copied images from the PACS environment and immediately transferring them to another server. By separating the nonclinical image server from the PACS server, we protect the clinical performance of the PACS. The availability of the PACS workstations is maximized, and the traffic on the PACS network is minimized. Our system also enhances access to the images because any computer on the network—not just the PACS workstations—can be used to manipulate and view the copied images.

manipulate [mə'nipjuleit] *v.* 操作、控制

第 64 天

学习

CT is an invaluable tool in the diagnosis of the chest diseases with high-resolution CT (HRCT) providing exquisite visualization of the pulmonary interstitium. However, CT examinations do not come without a cost. A report from the 2002 National Conference on Dose Reduction in CT indicates that CT now represents the largest single source of medical radiation exposure. Although CT constitutes only 15% of the total number of examinations in some university departments, it can account for 70% of the dose delivered.

在诊断胸部疾病时，CT 是一种极有价值的工具，高分辨率 CT（high-resolution CT，HRCT）可以提供肺间质的精细可视的图像。然而，做 CT 检查并不是没有代价的。一份 2002 年关于降低 CT 剂量的全国会议报告显示，CT 目前是医学辐射暴露接触最大的独立来源。虽然 CT 在大学科室中只占检查总数的 15%，但是却占放射剂量的 70%。

high-resolution CT 高分辨率 CT，简称 HRCT　　exquisite ['ekskwizit] *a.* 灵敏的

interstitium [intəs'tiʃəm] *n.* 间质组织

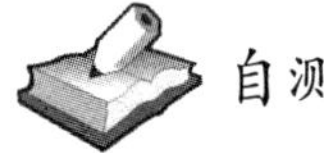
自测

之前已有几例研究报道在不同的放射诊断操作过程中的放射剂量以及给患者带来的相关风险。但是其中绝大多数研究针对的是成人患者，而儿童因放射曝光而导致癌致死概率预计高出成人每剂量单位的 2 ~ 4 倍，其原因尚未完全明确。但是儿童快速的细胞增殖速率和自身更长的平均寿命两者都造成其产生后遗效应的风险增加。因此，放射防护当局已经开始优先调查儿童的 X 线放射剂量水平和放射检查频率。其主要目的是能

够确定一个针对各项放射检查推荐的最大剂量值和能够满足仪器设备标准需求的最小剂量值。

答案

Several studies have been performed on dose and related risk to the patient from different diagnostic radiological procedures. The vast majority of these studies have concerned adult patients. However, the risk of lethal cancer from radiation exposure of children is expected to be 2-4 times higher than for adults per dose unit. The reason for this difference is not fully clear, but greater cell proliferation rate and longer life expectancy for children both result in a higher risk of developing late effects. Therefore, initiatives have been taken among radiation protection authorities to give priority to investigations of dose levels and frequencies of X-ray examinations among children. The main objective is to establish recommendations of upper dose limits for various diagnostic procedures and to implement minimum requirements for equipment standards.

lethal ['li:θl] *a.* 致死的　　vast [vɑ:st] *a.* 巨大的
majority [mə'dʒɔriti] *n.* 大部分　　initiative [i'niʃətiv] *a.* 初步的
priority [prai'ɔriti] *n.* 先前　　adult ['ædʌlt] *a.* 成人; *n.* 成人
expectancy [ik'spektənsi] *n.* 预期、期望
recommendation [ˌrekəmen'deiʃən] *n.* 建议、推荐
the recommendation is made that... 建议……

二、 交代研究意图

在阐述完大的学术背景后,紧接着要用简洁的语言交代作者所研究的意图,在此要直奔主题。

第 65 天

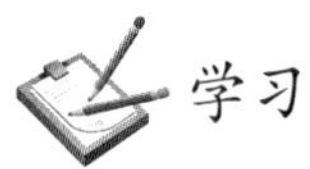
学习

In this study, the diagnostic performance of a digital large-area silicon flat-panel detector was compared with that of a conventional screen-film system in clinical chest imaging using abnormal findings documented by CT as the reference standard.

在本研究中,利用病案中 CT 发现的病灶作为参考标准,比较了数字大面积硅平板探测器与传统屏 - 片系统的临床胸部成像的诊断性能。

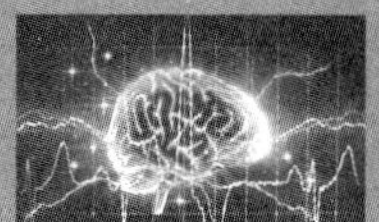

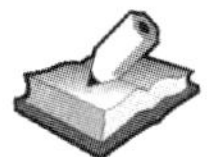 自测

在我们的研究中,我们采用一个全尺寸原型探测器在一小组患者中进行后前位胸部 X 线摄影,设法显示在影像质量下降未明显觉察时剂量下降的潜能。

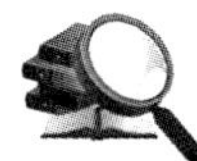 答案

In our study, we sought to show the potential for dose reduction without a perceivable loss of image quality for posteroanterior chest radiography on a small group of patients using a full-size prototype detector.

perceivable *a.* 可见的　　　prototype ['prəutətaip] *n.* 原型

第 66 天

 学习

We evaluated the image quality by using a large-area, solid-state X-ray detector based on the CsI/a-Si technique and studying routine chest images of the same patients obtained at different dose levels.

我们采用基于 CsI/a-Si 技术的大面积、固态 X 线探测器,通过研究在不同剂量水平获得同一患者的常规胸部影像,评价影像质量。

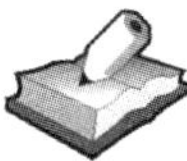 自测

在本研究中,我们分析了在系统日常运用过程中,出现在数字胸部影像中的记忆伪影,以及能使伪影的产生降到最低程度的方法。

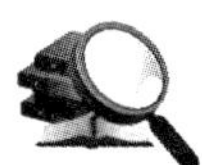 答案

In this study, we evaluated memory artifacts that can be seen in digital chest images acquired during routine system use, as well as methods that can be used to minimize their occurrence.

第 67 天

 学习

In this study, an observer test was performed to evaluate objectively the effect of the temporal subtraction images produced with this method on the detection of abnormalities in digital chest radiographs.

在此项研究中，在数字胸部X线摄片的异常诊断方面采用观察测试，对用这种方法产生的时间减影图像进行客观评价。

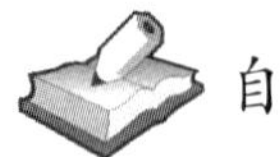
自测

在本篇文章中，我们描述当前放射摄影技术方面的研究状况，如传统胸部成像的应用，并讨论有关选择和应用市场上已有产品的实际问题。

答案

In this article we described the current state of the art in radiographic techniques as applied to routine thoracic imaging and discussed practical issues concerning the selection and use of commercially available products.

第 68 天

学习

The purpose of this study was to subjectively compare the image quality of 1-spr and 0.75-spr helical CT scans of the abdomen.

此项研究的目的是从主观上比较腹部螺旋 CT 扫描在 1 spr 和 0.75 spr 的影像质量。

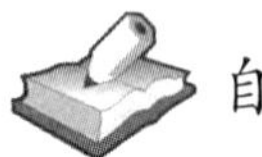
自测

下面我们谈谈在患者简单体位时，可采用螺旋扫描生成腕部直接冠状 CT 影像。

答案

We described a method for obtaining direct coronal CT images of the wrist using helical acquisition coupled with a simplified patient position.

第 69 天

学习

It was the purpose of this study to evaluate the influence of CT attenuation maps obtained

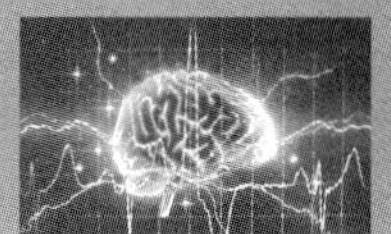

during deep respiration and normal end expiration on the quality of final attenuation-corrected PET images obtained in patients examined with a combined in-line PET/CT scanner.

这就是我们这次研究的目的：使用兼 PET / CT 为一体的扫描仪为患者做检查，评价在深呼吸过程中所获取的 CT 衰减影像和平静呼气末的 CT 衰减影像对最终所获得的衰减校正 PET 图像质量的影响。

attenuation[əˌtenju'eiʃən] *n.* 衰减　　　respiration[ˌrespə'reiʃn] *n.* 呼吸

expiration[ˌekspaiə'reiʃən] *n.* 呼出

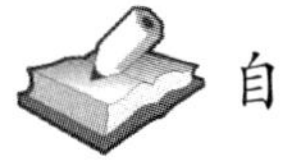

自测

因此，我们研究的目的是预测性评价 16 排探测器 CT 冠状动脉血管造影心率和图像重建技术对图像质量的影响。

答案

Thus, the aim of our study was to prospectively evaluate to what extent image quality in 16-detector row CT coronary angiography is a function of the heart rate and image reconstruction technique.

16-detector row CT　16 排探测器 CT

第 70 天

学习

The purpose of this study was to assess the technical feasibility of Xe ventilation CT with a DE technique by comparing it with simulated conventional CT in terms of measurement errors at dynamic quantification of Xe enhancement in the lung. We also obtained Xe ventilation CT images of the whole lung to compare them with simulated conventional CT images.

这项研究的目的是通过与模拟的常规 CT 在肺上 Xe 的动态增强的测量误差相比，评估拥有双能量技术的 Xe 通气 CT 在技术上的可行性。我们也获得了整个肺的 Xe 通气 CT 的图像，并用来和模拟的传统 CT 图像相比较。

ventilation[ˌventi'leiʃən] *n.* 通气　　　simulate['simjuleit] *vt.* 模拟

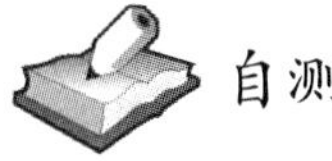

自测

我们的研究目标是预测性评估心率、心率的变化以及钙化对双源 CT 图像质量的影响，同时通过将有创冠状动脉血管造影作为参考标准，来初步评估双源 CT 对冠状动脉狭窄的诊断精度。

答案

The aim of our study was to prospectively evaluate the effect of heart rate, heart rate variability, and calcification on dual-source CT image quality and to prospectively assess the diagnostic accuracy of dual-source CT for coronary artery stenosis, by using invasive coronary angiography as the reference standard.

第 71 天

学习

Our study used a cohort design to evaluate the association between mammographic clinical image quality and the detection of cancer at the time of a screening visit.

我们的研究是用一组设计来评价普查时乳腺 X 线摄影临床影像质量与癌症探测之间的关系。

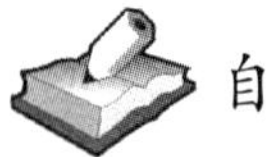

自测

本研究关注观片灯遮蔽和亮度在乳腺 X 线摄影方面的重要性。

答案

This work paid attention to the importance of viewbox masking and viewbox luminance levels in mammography.

第 72 天

学习

The purpose of our study was to determine the appearance of motion artifact using a digital slot-scanning system designed for mammography, taking timing and direction into account and using an anthropomorphic phantom to simulate clinical images.

我们研究的目的是测定采用数字裂隙扫描系统进行乳腺 X 线摄影时，移动伪影的表现，考虑时间和方向的因素，用仿真体模模拟临床影像。

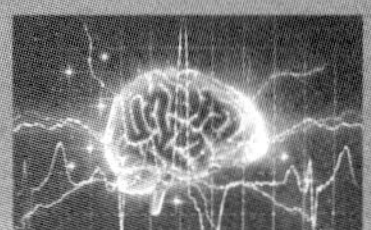

anthropomorphic *a.* 拟人的、类人的

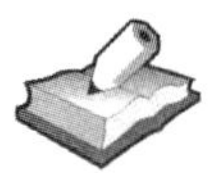 自测

本研究旨在比较以 CCD 为基础的数字乳腺 X 线摄影与传统乳腺 X 线摄影在各种不同的背景下病变的诊断力。

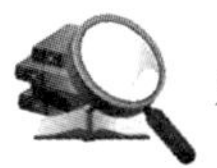 答案

The present study was performed to compare the lesion detectability between CCD-based digital mammography and conventional mammography under the various background.

第 73 天

 学习

The purpose of our study was, therefore, to compare the image quality of CRT display and LCD in a clinical setting by subjective assessment of the quality of side-by-side images.

因此，我们的研究目的是对 CRT 显示器和 LCD 的影像质量进行临床主观评价。

subjective assessment 主观评价

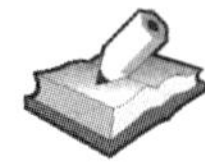 自测

此研究的目的是比较不同显示格式及不同观察系统的计算机 X 线照片对泌尿系结石的检出情况。

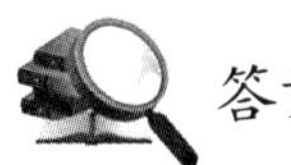 答案

The purpose of this study was to compare observer performance for the detection of urinary system calculi using computed radiographs with different display formats and different viewing systems.

第 74 天

 学习

The purpose of this study was to compare diagnostic performance, reviewer confidence, and time requirements in the MRI diagnosis of meniscal tears for three types of reviewers and two types of image documentation [soft copy (PACS) *vs* hard copy].

这个研究的目的是比较半月板撕裂的 MRI 诊断和两类图像存档 [软拷贝 (PACS) 和硬拷贝] 方面的诊断性能、读片者可信度及时间要求。

meniscal [mi'niskəl] *a.* 半月板的　　tear [tεə] *vt.* (tore, torn) 撕、损伤

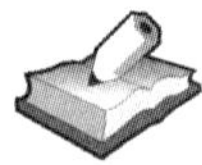 自测

本次研究的目的就是为了确定通过采用 5 mm 标准单螺旋胸部扫描和采用 1.25 mm HRCT 获得图像时，放射剂量是否降低。

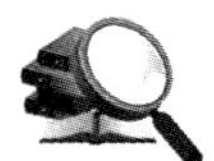 答案

The goal of this study was to determine if radiation exposure could be decreased by performing a single helical scan of the chest from which both 5-mm standard and 1.25-mm HRCT images could be obtained.

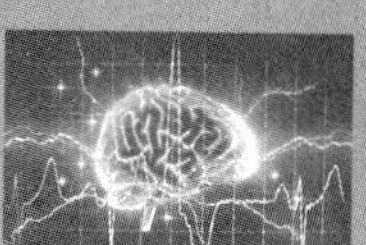

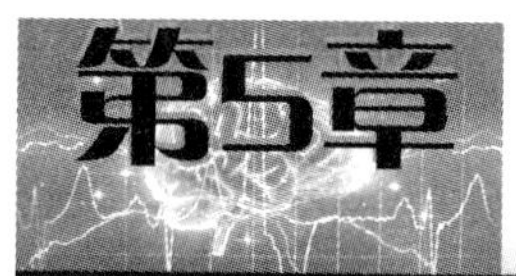

第5章　正文（Body）

在这一部分作者须阐述所采用的病例资料，具体使用的设备、应用的条件、评价的方法，以及采用什么统计学方法对数据进行处理，同时，也需要伦理委员会的同意或授权，甚至在这一段作者还可以适当地坦诚研究不足之处。

一、病例资料

病例资料应包括作者所使用病例的时间范围、年龄大小、男女例数、选择条件，以及不包含在内的理由等。

第 75 天

学习

We prospectively performed MR imaging in 50 healthy subjects: 21 men and 29 women (mean age, 60 years old; range, 23—84 years old).

我们按预期施行了 50 例健康人的 MR 成像调查：男性 21 例、女性 29 例（平均年龄 60 岁，年龄范围 23 ~ 84 岁）。

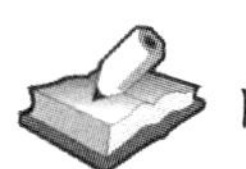

自测

最初筛选出的 114 幅影像，约一半采用数字软拷贝观察技术，另一半采用数字硬拷贝胶片。所有进行了排泄性尿路造影的患者 85 人，超声的 107 人，CT 的 79 人。

答案

The initial screening resulted in the selection of 114 images. Approximately half of these were selected using the digital soft-copy display as the viewing technique; the remaining half were selected using the digital hard-copy film during the screening. All patients underwent excretory urography ($n = 85$), sonography ($n = 107$), or CT ($n = 79$).

excretory [ek'skri:təri] *a.* 排泄的　　sonography [sə'nɔgrəfi] *n.* 超声检查

第 76 天

学习

From June to August 1998, 80 patients (46 men and 34 women; age range, 18—91 years old; mean age, 63 years old) from different clinical departments who underwent CT and radiography of the chest with a conventional screen-film system were examined. All patients had one or more radiographic abnormalities. All examinations were performed within 48 hr.

从 1998 年 6 月至 8 月，来自不同临床科室的 80 例患者（男性 46 例、女性 34 例；年龄 18 ~ 91 岁；平均年龄 63 岁）进行了胸部 CT 及传统屏 - 片系统的 X 线摄影检查。在 X 线照片上所有患者都存在 1 个或更多的异常。所有检查在 48 小时内完成。

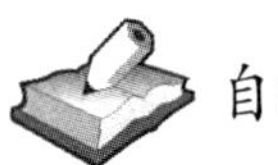

自测

从 21 岁以上的患者中随机选择志愿者进行四肢成像。患者年龄范围为 50 ~ 80 岁。患者 X 线摄影诊断包括正常、骨折、关节炎、既往外科手术及缺血性坏死。

答案

Volunteers were selected randomly from the patients older than 21 years old referred for imaging of the extremities. Patients' ages ranged from 50 to 80. Patients' radiographic diagnoses included normal, fracture, arthritis, previous surgery, and avascular necrosis.

extremity [ik'streməti] 末端，肢　　fracture ['fræktʃə] *n.* 骨折

arthritis [ɑ:'θraitis] *n.* 关节炎；复数 arthritides [ɑ:'θritidi:z]

avascular [ə'væskjulə] *a.* 无血管的

necrosis [ne'krəusis] *n.* 坏死；复数 necroses [ne'krəusi:z]

volunteer [vɔlən'tiə] *n.* 志愿者；volunteer to... 自愿做……

randomly *ad.* 随机地

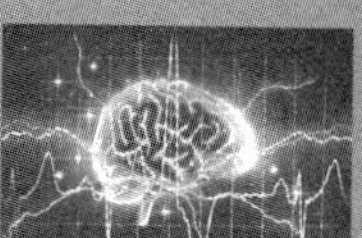

第 77 天

学习

Using our radiology information system software, we randomly selected 50 patients (24 women, 26 men; age range, 16—79 years old; mean age, 57 years old) who had chest radiographs obtained in posteroanterior and lateral projections during both the period in which the detector dose was 2.5 μGy and the period in which the dose was 1.8 μGy. In cases of multiple available studies, the studies with the shortest time elapsed between them were used for further evaluation (interval range, 13—73 days; mean interval, 41 days).

采用我们的放射信息系统软件，我们随机选择获得胸部后前位和侧位摄影 X 线照片的 50 例患者（24 例女性，26 例男性；年龄范围 16 ~ 79 岁，平均年龄 57 岁），既有 2.5 μGy 探测器剂量期间的，又有 1.8 μGy 探测器剂量期间的患者。就这么多可得到的研究而言，我们对在它们中用最短时间阅片进行进一步评价（间隔范围 13 ~ 73 天，平均间隔 41 天）。

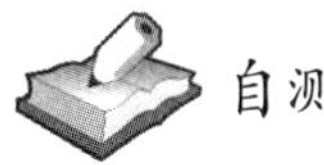
自测

肺部异常的临床诊断或拟诊不影响对患者的选择。此研究包括正常患者的 X 线照片（2.5 μGy 的 6 例，1.8 μGy 的 7 例）和患病者的 X 线照片，如胸腔积液、气胸、肺炎、肺结节和肺不张，以及伴有如胸管、中心静脉导管或起搏器等异物的患者（2.5 μGy 的 44 例，1.8 μGy 的 43 例）。

答案

Clinical diagnosis or expectation of certain pulmonary abnormalities did not influence patient selection. The studies included both radiographs of patients with normal findings (n = 6 obtained at 2.5 μGy, n = 7 obtained at 1.8 μGy) and patients with diseases such as pleural effusion, pneumothorax, pneumonia, lung nodules, and atelectasis as well as those with foreign bodies like chest tubes, central venous catheters, or pacemaker (n = 44 obtained at 2.5 μGy, n = 43 obtained at 1.8 μGy).

pulmonary ['pʌlmənəri] *a.* 肺的

effusion [i'fju:ʒən] *n.* 渗出、渗出液

pneumothorax [ˌnju:məu'θɔ:ræks] *n.* 气胸

lung [lʌŋ] *n.* 肺

atelectasis [ˌætə'lektəsis] *n.* 肺不张

catheter ['kæθitə] *n.* 导管

pleural *a.* 胸膜的

pleural effusion 胸腔积液

pneumonia [nju(:)'məunjə] *n.* 肺炎

nodule ['nɔdju:l] *n.* 结、小结

venous ['vi:nəs] *a.* 静脉的

pacemaker ['peismeikə] *n.* 起搏器

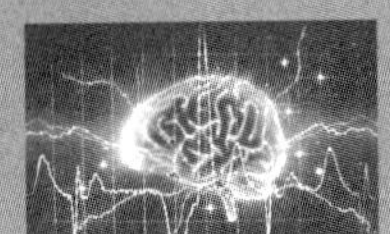

第 78 天

学习

In a prospective study, 70 patients (49 men, 21 women) consecutively underwent multi-detector row CT coronary angiography. Of these patients, 49 (33 men, 16 women) also underwent invasive coronary angiography. The mean time between examinations was 23 days (range, 13—39 days). The average age of patients was 59.1 years old (age range, 29—65 years old), and the mean heart rate was 70.7 beats per minute (range, 45—105 beats per minute).

在一项前瞻性的研究中，70 例（男 49，女 21）进行了多排探测器 CT 冠状动脉造影。在这些患者中，49 例（男 33，女 16）同时进行了有创冠状动脉造影。平均检查时间为 23 天（范围为 13 ~ 39 天）。患者平均年龄是 59.1 岁（年龄范围为 29 ~ 65 岁），平均心率为 70.7/min（范围为 45 ~ 105/min）。

prospective [prəs'pektiv] *a.* 未来的、预期的

multi-detector row CT 多排探测器 CT

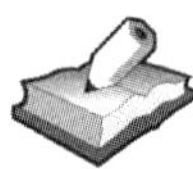

自测

找出 2001 年 3 月至 2003 年 3 月根据医院的电子图表因被怀疑有半月板撕裂而做了 MRI 检查的 120 例有编号的患者（55 例女性和 65 例男性；平均年龄：45.4 岁；年龄范围：16 ~ 80 岁）。只有当关节腔镜检查前未超过 4 个月做 MRI 检查和 MRI 检查前未做外科手术的患者才被列入这个研究。在这前提下 120 例患者中只有 71 例继续留在这项研究中。

答案

One hundred and twenty consecutive patients (55 women and 65 men; mean age, 45.4 years old; age range, 16—80 years old) with MRI examinations performed because of suspected meniscal tears were identified in the hospital's electronic charts between March 2001 and March 2003. These patients were included in this study only when MRI was performed no longer than 4 months before arthroscopy and when no surgery had been performed before MRI. After application of these criteria, 71 of the original 120 patients remained in the study.

meniscal [mi'niskəl] *a.* 半月板的　　tear [tɛə] *vt.* 撕、损伤

arthroscopy [ɑ:'θrɔskəpi] *n.* 关节镜检查

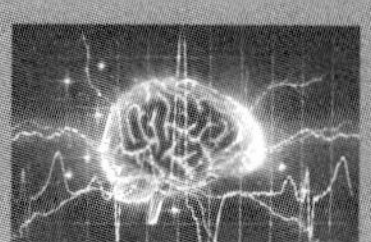

第 79 天

学习

All examinations were performed between October 2002 and November 2003. A total of 49 patients underwent multi-detector row CT coronary angiography before minimally invasive bypass surgery for planning purposes; 21 patients underwent multi-detector row CT coronary angiography because of intermediate pretest likelihood of coronary artery disease, although they had symptomatic chest pain. Included were patients who had a regular heart rate during scanning (ie, the difference between the minimum and maximum value was ＜ 15 beats per minute). Exclusion criteria were the presence of coronary artery stent, absolute tachyarrhythmia, difference of more than 15 beats per minute between the minimum and maximum heart rate, hypersensitivity to iodinated contrast media, renal failure (serum creatinine level ＞ 100 mmol/L), pregnancy, respiratory impairment, or pronounced cardiac failure.

检查时间为 2002 年 10 月到 2003 年 11 月。共有 49 例患者在进行微创介入手术前做了多排探测器 CT 冠状动脉造影；21 例胸痛疑有冠心病的患者接受了多排探测器 CT 冠状动脉造影。列入研究的患者在扫描期间的心率很规律（其最低和最高值相差＜ 15/min）。患者不存在以下情况：冠状动脉扩张、绝对性心律失常、最高最低心率差异＞ 15/min、对碘对比剂过敏、肾衰竭（血清肌酐水平＞ 100 mmol/L）、怀孕、呼吸障碍或明显的心脏衰竭。

coronary artery stent 冠状动脉扩张　　absolute tachyarrhythmia 绝对性心律失常

hypersensitivity [ˌhaipə(:)ˌsensə'tivəti] *n.* 过敏反应、超敏反应

renal failure 肾衰竭　　serum creatinine level 血清肌酐水平

pregnancy ['pregnənsi] *n.* 妊娠、怀孕　　respiratory impairment 呼吸障碍

pronounced [prə'naunst] *a.* 显著的、明显的

cardiac failure 心脏衰竭　　symptomatic [simptə'mætik] *a.* 有症状的

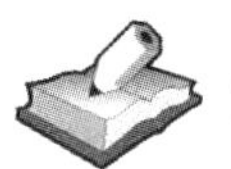

自测

在 4 个月中，我们通过数字平板探测器 X 线摄影系统对 112 例无症状的患者摄片，并获得后前位和侧位胸部 X 线照片。所有患者来自当地肿瘤外科临床门诊，且被常规随访检查。所有患者在用数字系统实际检查前 1 年内都做了后前位和侧位屏 - 片胸部 X 线照片（平均 192 天，最短 34 天，最长 365 天）。影像评价前，我们对所有硬拷贝在两次检查中胸部解剖的变化做了判断（如由治疗或肺部疾病所造成的变化）。3 例患者因为胸部手术导致解剖的改变而被排除在这项研究之外。所有其他患者显示正常。另外，有 9 例患者在影像评价时由于屏 - 片图像被借到其他医院，故也不包括在本研究中。

答案

In a 4-month period, posteroanterior and lateral chest radiographs were obtained from 112 consecutive asymptomatic patients using a digital flat-panel detector radiography system. All patients were from the outpatient oncology clinics of the local surgery department and were examined for a routine follow-up. All patients had previous posteroanterior and lateral film-screen chest radiographs within a period of 1 year (mean, 192 days; minimum, 34 days; maximum, 365 days) before the actual examination with the digital system. Before the image evaluation, all hard copies were checked for changes in the chest anatomy (e.g., changes resulting from therapy or pulmonary disease) between the two examinations. Three patients were excluded from the study because of alterations of the chest anatomy caused by thoracic surgery. All other patients showed normal findings. Another nine patients were excluded from the study because the film-screen images were on loan to other hospitals at the time of image evaluation.

consecutive [kən'sekjutiv] *a.* 连续的

a digital flat-panel detector radiography system 数字平板探测器 X 线摄影系统

outpatient ['autˌpeiʃənt] *n.* 门诊病人

oncology [ɔŋ'kɔlədʒi] *n.* 肿瘤学

surgery ['sə:dʒəri] *n.* 外科、外科学

follow-up ['fɔləuˌʌp] *n.* 随访

actual ['æktjuəl] *a.* 实际的、事实上

anatomy [ə'nætəmi] *n.* 解剖学、解剖

therapy ['θerəpi] *n.* 治疗

thoracic [θɔ:'ræsik] *a.* 胸的、胸廓的

第 80 天

学习

Helical CT scans of the abdomen and pelvis were obtained in 37 patients. Seventeen scans were obtained consecutively using 0.75-spr scanning, and 20 scans were obtained consecutively using 1.0-spr scanning. There were nine women and eight men in the 0.75-spr group and 11 women and 9 men in the 1.0-spr group. The mean ages for the 0.75- and 1.0-spr groups were 58 years old (range：30—75 years old) and 59 years old (range:34—92 years old), respectively. The indications for the CT scans included staging of known primary tumor (16), abdominal pain (3), cirrhosis (pretransplant evaluation) (2), abdominal mass (2), small bowel obstruction (1), thoracoabdominal aneurysm (1), pancreatitis (1),and fever (1). Each patient received 150ml of either iohexol 240 or diatrizoate meglumine 60% IV contrast material. Eight of 17 patients in the 0.75-spr group and 4 of 20 patients in the 1.0-spr group received nonionic contrast material.

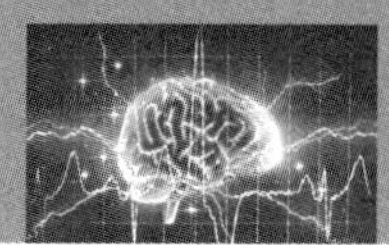

腹部和盆腔螺旋 CT 扫描 37 例。17 例采用 0.75 spr 连续扫描，20 例采用 1.0 spr 连续扫描。在 0.75 spr 一组中女性 9 例、男性 8 例，在 1.0 spr 一组中女性 11 例、男性 9 例。0.75 spr 组和 1.0 spr 组的平均年龄分别是 58 岁（范围：30 ～ 75 岁）、59 岁（范围：34 ～ 92 岁）。CT 扫描的指征包括已知原发肿瘤（16 例）、腹痛（3 例）、硬化（移植前评价）（2 例）、腹部肿块（2 例）、小肠梗阻（1 例）、胸腹部动脉瘤（1 例）、胰腺炎（1 例）以及发热（1 例）。每例患者静脉注射 150 ml 碘海醇 240 或 60% 泛影葡胺对比剂。在 0.75 spr 一组中 17 例患者中的 8 例和在 1.0 spr 一组中 20 例患者中的 4 例接受非离子型对比剂。

helical［'helikl］*a.* 螺旋的
scan［skæn］*v.* 扫描
pelvis［'pelvis］*n.* 骨盆；复数 pelvises 或 pelves
primary［'praiməri］*a.* 原发的
tumor［'tju:mə］*n.* 肿瘤
cirrhosis［si'rəusis］*n.* 硬变
small bowel 小肠
obstruction［əb'strʌkʃən］*n.* 梗阻
aneurysm［'ænjuərizəm］*n.* 动脉瘤
pancreatitis［ˌpæŋkriə'taitis］*n.* 胰腺炎
iohexol［ˌaiəu'heksɔl］*n.* 碘海醇
diatrizoate meglumine 泛影葡胺
nonionic contrast material 非离子型对比剂

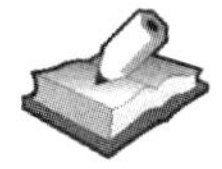

自测

从 2006 年 9 月到 2007 年 3 月我们扫描了 119 例患者，这些患者是准备进行有创冠状动脉血管造影的，因为他们被怀疑有冠心病或者病情有进展。排除对象包括：肾功能不全者（血清肌酐水平 ＞ 132.6 μmol/L），甲状腺功能亢进症者（基础甲状腺类激素 ＜ 0.03 μl/L），对碘对比剂过敏的和不能根据指示控制呼吸者。排除做过血管旁路手术的患者，而行冠状动脉旁路移植术者则留下。8 例拒绝的或者反悔的患者没有参加本次研究。2 例肾功能不全的和 7 例之前行冠状动脉旁路的以及 1 例因急性冠状动脉综合征须紧急行有创冠状动脉造影的患者也被排除在外。在进行了冠状动脉 CT 血管造影后有一个患者拒绝再进行有创冠状动脉造影。因此，本次研究的最终人数是 100（20 例女性，80 例男性；平均年龄为 62 岁 ± 10 岁）。75 例患者正接受 β 受体阻滞药的基本治疗。不允许做超量 β 受体阻滞药的治疗。所有的双源 CT 均在有创冠状动脉造影的前一天进行。

答案

From September 2006 to March 2007 we screened 119 patients who were scheduled to undergo invasive coronary angiography because they were suspected of having coronary artery disease or the progression of known coronary artery disease was suspected. Exclusion criteria were renal insufficiency (serum creatinine level ＞ 132.6 μmol/L), hyperthyroidism (basal thyroid-stimulating hormone ＜ 0.03 μl/L), known allergic reaction to iodinated contrast medium, and inability to follow breath-hold commands. Patients who underwent bypass surgery were excluded from this study, while patients with coronary artery bypass grafting were not. Eight patients could not be enrolled because of the refusal or withdrawal of consent. Two patients were excluded because of impaired renal function, seven were excluded because of previous bypass surgery, and one was excluded because of acute coronary syndrome necessitating immediate invasive coronary angiography. After coronary CT angiography, one patient declined to undergo invasive coronary angiography. Thus, the ultimate study population comprised 100 patients (20 women, 80 men; mean age, 62 years old ± 10). Seventy-five of these patients were taking a beta-blocker as part of their baseline medication. Additional beta-blocker medication was not administered. All dual-source CT studies were performed the day prior to invasive coronary angiography.

renal insufficiency 肾功能不全
hyperthyroidism [ˌhaipə(:)'θairɔidizəm] *n.* 甲状腺功能亢进症
schedule ['ʃedju:l] *vt.* 计划；be scheduled to 预备做某事
basal thyroid-stimulating hormone 基础促甲状腺激素
allergic [ə'lə:dʒik] *a.* 过敏性的、变应性的
withdrawal [wið'drɔ:əl] *n.* 收回、撤销
acute coronary syndrome 急性冠状动脉综合征
refusal [ri'fju:zl] *n.* 拒绝
consent [kən'sent] *v.* 同意
beta-blocker β 受体阻滞药

二、 应用设备

此段须阐述作者所使用的仪器设备、生产厂商、机器型号。

第 81 天

All studies were performed on a 1.0-T MR imager.
所有研究用 1.0T MR 成像仪完成。

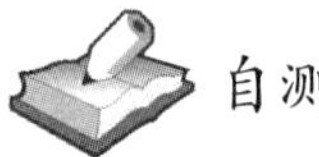

后前位及侧位胸部 X 线照片是利用数字系统获得的。

Posteroanterior and lateral chest radiographs were obtained with a digital system.

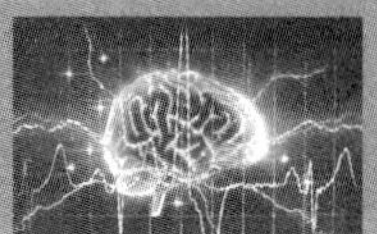

第 82 天

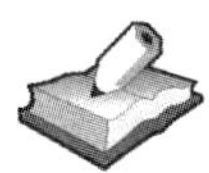
学习

Images were transferred to a laser imager to be printed on laser films (35 cm × 43 cm).

影像被传递给激光成像仪打印在激光胶片上（35 cm × 43 cm）。

laser film 激光胶片

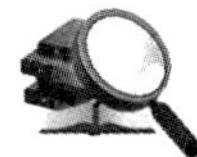
自测

使用一种新型平板探测器系统完成患者立位的胸部数字 X 线摄影。

答案

A new flat-panel detector system was used to perform the digital chest radiography with the patient in an erect position.

an erect position 立位

第 83 天

学习

We used a standard X-ray tube and a standard high-voltage generator; the automatic exposure control was adjusted to a 400-speed class. The system included a moving grid (40 line pairs per centimeter; ratio = 12).

我们采用标准 X 线管及标准高压发生器；将自动曝光控制调至 400 速度级。此系统包括一个活动滤线栅（40 lp/cm, 栅比 =12）。

X-ray tube　X 线管　　high-voltage generator 高压发生器

automatic exposure control 自动曝光控制　　moving grid 活动滤线栅

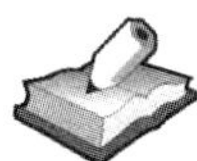
自测

MRI 应用 1.0T（n=30 例患者）或 1.5T（n=41 例患者）进行扫描。两个系统均使用偏振线圈，发射 - 接收四肢线圈。

答案

MRI was performed on either a 1.0-T magnet (n = 30 patients) or a 1.5-T magnet (n = 41 patients) on the basis of the availability of the scanners. A dedicated circularly polarized, send-receive extremity coil was used on both systems.

polarized *a*. 极化的、偏振的

第 84 天

学习

The detector has a matrix size of 2048 × 2048 pixels, with a pixel size of 200 μm. The active area that the detector measures is 41 cm × 41 cm. The maximum spatial resolution achieved with this detector is 2.5 line pairs per millimeter. The digital radiography system also included a standard X-ray tube and a standard high-voltage 80-kW generator.

此探测器矩阵为 2 048 × 2 048，像素为 200 μm。探测器测试的实际区域为 41 cm × 41 cm。此探测器的最大空间分辨率达到 2.5 lp/mm。数字 X 线摄影系统也包括标准的 X 线管和标准 80 kW 的高压发生器。

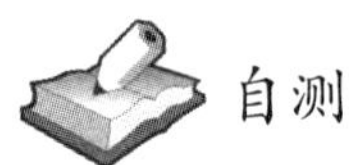

自测

此系统由 X 线管（焦点大小为 0.6 mm 和 1.0 mm）、直立屏风、固定滤线栅（80 lp/cm，栅比 15∶1），和安装在曝光感受器、滤线栅和碳纤维盘之后的平板 CsI/a-Si 探测器组成。此系统的探测器焦距为 180 cm。矩阵大小为 3 000 × 3 000，像素 143 μm × 143 μm，实际成像区域 43 cm × 43 cm，理论上的空间分辨率为 3.5 lp/mm。

答案

The system consisted of an X-ray tube (focal spot sizes, 0.6 mm and 1.0 mm), a wall stand, a stationary grid (80 line pairs centimeter, ratio 15 : 1), and the flat-panel CsI/a-Si detector mounted behind the phototimer sensor, grid, and carbon fibre plate. Detector-focus distance of the system was 180 cm. Matrix size was 3 000 × 3 000 with a pixel size of 143 μm × 143 μm, leading to an active imaging area of 43 cm × 43 cm and a theoretical limit of spatial resolution of 3.5 line pairs per millimeter.

focal spot size 焦点大小

stationary grid 固定滤线栅

phototimer ['fəutəutaimə] *n*. 曝光计

sensor ['sensə] *n*. 传感器、感受器

carbon ['kɑ:bən] *n*. 碳

fibre ['faibə*r*] *n*. 纤维

detector-focus distance 探测器与焦点之间的距离

theoretical [θiə'retikəl] *a*. 理论上的

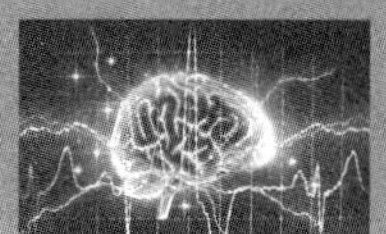

第 85 天

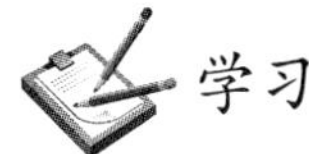
学习

All studies were performed with a combined PET/CT in-line system that enables the acquisition of CT and PET data in the same patient in one session. The axes of both systems are mechanically aligned to allow for “hardware” image co-registration.

所有这些研究都是由兼 PET/CT 于一体的系统来完成的。该系统可以使 CT 和 PET 的数据采集在同一患者身上、在同一时间内进行。为了使硬件图像记录系统协同地进行，2 套系统的轴线在机械上紧密地结合。

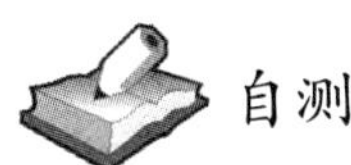
自测

使用 6 台 CT（A-F）进行 CT SPR。在此研究中使用下列 CT 扫描仪：A 为多排探测器螺旋 CT，GE 公司 QX/ Ⅰ 型；B 为单排探测器螺旋 CT，GE 公司 CT/ Ⅰ 型；C 为单排探测器螺旋 CT，GE 公司 Hi Speed/RP 型；D 为非螺旋 CT，GE 公司 9800 型；E 为电子束 CT，Imatron 公司 C150-XLPHRD 型；F 为单排探测器螺旋 CT，Picker 公司 PQ6000 型。

答案

Six CT systems (A to F) were used to perform CT SPR . The following CT scanners were used in this study: system A, multi-detector row spiral CT, model QX/ Ⅰ , GE Medical Systems; system B, single-detector row spiral CT, model CT/ Ⅰ , GE Medical Systems; system C, single-detector row spiral CT, model Hi Speed/RP, GE Medical Systems; system D, non-spiral CT, model 9800, GE Medical Systems; system E, electron-beam CT, model C150-XLPHRD, Imatron; system F, single-detector row spiral CT, model PQ6000, Picker.

multi-detector row spiral CT　多排探测器螺旋 CT
single-detector row spiral CT　单排探测器螺旋 CT
non-spiral CT　非螺旋 CT　　electron-beam CT　电子束 CT

三、 技术参数

要阐明作者在科研过程中所使用的一些体位与技术参数，如成像参数：千伏、毫安、秒、焦 - 片距、扫描层厚、层间距、重建算法、窗水平，以及作者在试验中所用的方法。

第 86 天

1. Exposure specifications were 125 kVp and a 200-cm film-focus distance.
   曝光条件为 125 kVp,焦 - 片距 200 cm。
   film-focus distance 焦 - 片距,也称 FFD
2. Posteroanterior and lateral radiographs were obtained with the patient in an erect position.
   患者取站立位获得后前位及侧位 X 线影像。

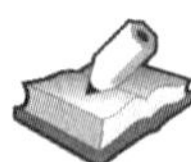

此技术可获得 5.6 lp/mm 的空间分辨率。在检查过程中使用了活动滤线栅(40 lp/cm,栅比= 12)。

The spatial resolution that can be achieved with this technique is 5.6 line pairs per millimeter. A moving grid (40 lines per centimeter; ratio = 12) was used.

第 87 天

1. Exposure specifications were set to be similar to those used to obtain the digital radiographs (e.g., 400-speed class, 125 kVp, and 200 cm film-focus distance), leading to comparable radiation doses for both methods.

采用曝光条件类似于获得数字 X 线照片的条件(如:速度 400、125 kVp、200 cm 焦 - 片距),确保两种方式运用相似的 X 线剂量。

2. A dose of 2.5 μGy corresponds to the dose that would be used with a 400-speed screen-film system. Thus, a detector dose of 1.8μGy results in a calculated speed of 560.

2.5 μGy 的剂量相当于使用 400 速度屏 - 片系统的剂量。因此 1.8 μGy 的探测器剂量相当于使用 560 速度屏 - 片系统的剂量。

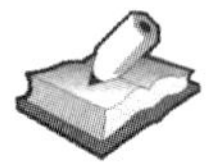

1. CT 研究使用的是 1 台双源 CT 扫描机,而且这些患者没有并发症。在获取 top 像之

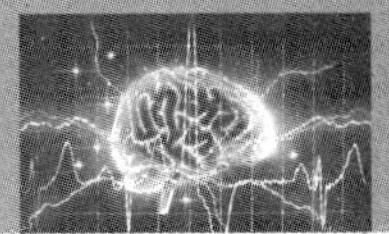

前，患者被单次注入了 2.5 mg 的碘剂。

2. 分别用硒数字 X 线摄影系统及传统速度为 100 的屏 - 片系统获得 25 对单个的手足影像。所有影像在台面上获得，未使用滤线栅，所有影像彼此在连续的几分钟内、在同一 X 线机房获得。

答案

1. CT studies were performed with a dual-source CT scanner in all patients and were performed without complications. Prior to acquisition of the topogram, patients received a single dose of 2.5 mg of idodine.

complication [ˌkɔmpli'keiʃən] *n.* 并发症　　prior ['praiə] *a.* 在前的（to）

topogram *n.* top 像

2. Twenty-five paired single images of the hand or foot were obtained with both the selenium-based digital radiography system and a conventional 100-speed film-screen system. All images were obtained on the tabletop without the use of an antiscatter grid, and all images were obtained in the same radiography room sequentially within several minutes of each other.

an antiscatter grid 防散射滤线栅

第 88 天

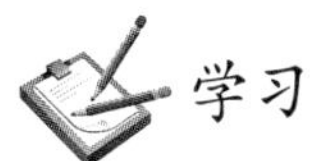

学习

An identical manual radiographic technique was used for both selenium-based digital radiographic images and conventional film-screen images. Manual exposures ranged from 46 to 66 kVp and from 3.2 to 6.3 mAs. Identical radiographic techniques were used to allow comparison of subjective image quality at the same radiation dose.

对于硒数字 X 线摄影影像及传统屏 - 片成像，采用同一的 X 线手动摄影技术进行操作。手动曝光范围为 46 ~ 66 kVp 及 3.2 ~ 6.3 mAs。使用相同的 X 线摄影技术在同一 X 线剂量下进行影像质量的主观比较。

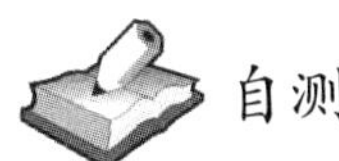

自测

总体钙化程度是通过使用原始的非增强 CT 扫描获得：准直器 32 mm × 0.6 mm；使用 Z 轴飞焦点技术获得层厚：64 mm × 0.6 mm；机架旋转时间：330 ms；螺距：0.2 ~ 0.39，取决于心率；管电流：80 mAs/r；管电压：120 kV。

答案

Total calcium burden was assessed by using an initial unenhanced CT scan with the following parameters: collimation, 32 mm × 0.6 mm; section acquisition, 64 mm × 0.6 mm with the Z-flying focal spot technique; gantry rotation time, 330 ms; pitch, 0.2—0.39, depending on heart rate; tube current, 80 mAs per rotation; and tube voltage, 120 kV.

burden ['bə:dn] *n.* 负担　　flying focal spot technique 飞焦点技术

第 89 天

学习

For contrast material-enhanced studies, vessel opacification was achieved by using automatic injection of 80 ml of iomeprol at a flow rate of 5ml/s and a 60-ml chaser bolus. Estimation of individual circulation time was based on the test-bolus technique, by using a 20-ml bolus and dynamic evaluation software.

在对比剂增强研究中，管腔充盈是通过自动注射 80ml 的碘对比剂、在 5ml/s 的流速和追加团注 60ml 生理盐水的条件下获得。个体循环时间的估计是基于弹丸测试技术，使用 20ml 的团注量和动态评价软件。

vessel ['vesl] *n.* 脉管　　opacification [əupæsifi'keiʃən] *n.* 不透光

flow rate 流率　　chaser ['tʃeisə] *n.* 追逐者

individual circulation time 个体循环时间

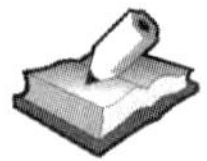

自测

在各例中做矢状位 T_1 加权像（重复时间 520 ms，回波时间 15 ms），层厚 7 mm，层间距 0.7 mm，矩阵 192 × 256，并获取 2 次信号。

答案

In each subject, sagittal T_1-weighted imaging (repetition time, 520 ms; echo time, 15 ms) was performed with 7mm thick sections, 0.7mm intersection gap, 192 × 256 matrix, and two signals acquired.

T_1-weighted imaging　T_1 加权成像　　thick section 厚层

repetition time 重复时间　　echo time 回波时间

intersection gap 层间距

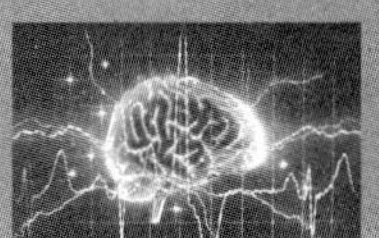

第 90 天

Film-screen radiography—as a standard reference, a 200-speed conventional film-screen system was used in this study. The conventional chest radiography system consisted of an automatic film changer, a standard X-ray tube, and a high-voltage 70 kW generator. The system worked with an automatic exposure control using 125 kVp for the posteroanterior and lateral radiographs. The film-focus distance was 220 cm. A moving grid (40 line pairs per centimeter; ratio, 12 : 1) was used.

屏 - 片 X 线摄影——根据参考标准，在本研究中使用 200 速度传统屏 - 片系统。传统胸部 X 线摄影系统由自动换片仪、标准 X 线管、70 kW 高压发生器组成。此系统采用了 125 kVp 的自动曝光控制对后前位和侧位进行 X 线摄片。焦 - 片距为 220 cm。使用活动滤线栅（40 lp/cm，栅比 12 : 1）。

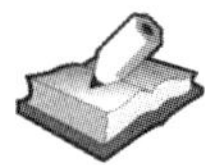

自测

用 8 mm 准直进行胸部螺旋 CT 扫描，床速 10 mm/s，重建间隙 8 mm。曝光参数为 1 s 扫描时间、137 kVp 和 145 mA。用高压注射器以 2 ml/s 的速率静脉注射 60 ml 非离子型对比剂（碘帕醇或碘普胺 300）。影像重建采用软组织算法，采用纵隔窗（窗宽 240 HU；窗位 60 HU）和肺窗（窗宽 2 000 HU，窗位 −500 HU）显示。

Helical CT of the chest was performed with an 8 mm collimation, a table speed of 10 mm/s, and 8 mm reconstruction intervals. Exposure parameters were 137 kVp and 145 mA with a 1 sec scan time. Sixty milliliters of IV nonionic contrast material [iopromide (Ultravist 300)] was administered by power injection at a rate of 2 ml/sc. Images were reconstructed using a soft-tissue algorithm and were displayed at mediastinal window settings (width, 240 HU; level, 60 HU) and at lung window settings (width, 2 000 HU; level, −500 HU).

reconstruction interval 重建间距
nonionic contrast material 非离子型对比剂
soft-tissue algorithm 软组织算法
mediastinal window 纵隔窗
lung window 肺窗

第 91 天

学习

The patient is positioned at the head of the CT scanner with his or her arm resting on the CT table parallel to the gantry. The patient is told to maintain that position while the table moves a short distance and is instructed to move his or her body with the table but not to resist the table motion. The patient is asked to look away from the gantry to minimize corneal radiation exposure. No additional stabilizing devices (such as pillows or tape) are typically required.

患者置于 CT 扫描仪的前端，将手臂自然地放在 CT 床面上，平行于机架。要求患者当床面移动一短距离时保持原位置不动，并告知他（或她）的身体随床面移动，但不能阻碍床面移动。要求患者不要看机架以减少角膜放射线曝光。不需要附加固定设备（诸如垫子或带子）。

corneal *a.* 角膜的
pillow ['piləu] *n.* 垫枕
stabilize ['steibəlaiz] *vt.* 使稳定
instruct [in'strʌkt] *vt.* 讲授、说明
resist [ri'zist] *v.* 阻碍

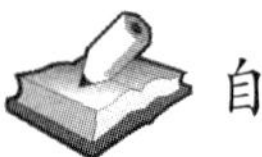

自测

本学院诊断性 MRI（用 1.5T 全身机）患者采取俯卧位，用双侧乳腺表面线圈和横向 T_1 加权二维快速小角度激发成像序列（重复时间 / 回波时间 = 200/5；翻转角，80°），静脉注射 0.1 mmol/kg 钆喷酸二甲基葡胺（前后获得 3 次诊断性 MR 图像），每序列时间为 1 min 46 s，层厚为 4 mm，层间距 5 mm，扫描野 350 mm，矩阵 256 × 256。恶性病变标准为早期对比剂增强，以后有一平稳期或信号强度缓慢降低。

答案

Diagnostic MR images in our institution (1.5-T whole body imager) are performed with the patient in the prone position, with use of a bilateral breast surface coil and a transverse T_1-weighted two-dimensional fast low-angle shot sequence (repetition time /echo time = 200/5; flip angle, 80°) before and three times after intravenous injection of 0.1 mmol/kg of gadopentetate dimeglumine.Time per sequence was 1 minute 46 seconds. The section thickness was 4 mm with a 1 mm gap (field of view, 350 mm; matrix, 256 × 256). Criteria for malignancy were the enhancement a initial strong contrast material with a subsequent plateau phase or a slow decrease in signal intensity.

bilateral [bai'lætərəl] *a.* 两侧的
prone [prəun] *a.* 易于……的（to）
fast low-angle shot sequence 快速小角度激发脉冲序列

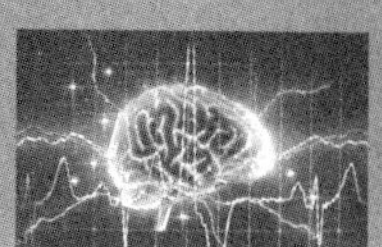

flip angle 翻转角　　intravenous injection 静脉注射
plateau [plæ'təu] *n.* 平高线、平顶；复数 plateaus 或 plateaux
field of view 视野，简称 FOV

第 92 天

学习

An FCR-9000 unit was used to obtain direct digital projectional radiographic images. We used 14inch × 17inch (36 cm × 43 cm) ST-V imaging plates (202 μm/pixel) with a matrix of 1 760 × 2 140 × 10 bit and a pixel size of 0.2 mm. Each storage phosphor image was 2MB. Images were then laser-printed onto film using an 80 μm spot, 12bit high-resolution laser printer. The printing procedure resulted in a 9.3% reduction in image size compared with the conventional radiographs.

采用 FCR-9000 型获得直接数字摄影 X 线照片影像。我们用 14 in × 17 in（36 cm × 43 cm）ST-V 成像板（每像素 202 μm），1 760 × 2 140 × 10 bit 的矩阵，每个像素大小为 0.2 mm。各个存储荧光影像为 2 MB。影像采用 80 μm 的点，12 bit 的高分辨率激光打印机打印胶片。影像尺寸与传统 X 线照片相比因打印操作而减小了 9.3%。

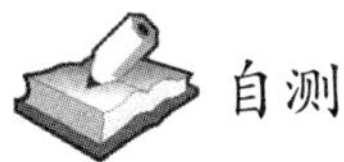

自测

我们使用平板数字 X 线摄影系统获取后前位胸部 X 线照片。曝光条件采用 125 kVp，栅比 12 : 1，探测器球管距离 2 mm，400 感度调制的自动曝光控制。我们科在常规进行胸部照片硬拷贝处理时通常采用同样算法，这种算法基于非锐利卷积滤过（肺相应的光学密度为 1.8，灰度系数 2.6，细节对比增强 0.4，噪声衰减 0.8）。影像矩阵为 2 941 × 3 021，每个像素大小为 0.143 mm。

答案

We obtained the posteroanterior chest radiographs with a flat-panel digital radiography system. Exposures were taken with 125 kVp, an integrated 12 : 1 grid, and a 2 mm detector–tube distance using automatic exposure control that was adjusted to a system sensitivity of 400. Images were processed with the same algorithm that is routinely used in our institution for processing hard copies of chest films and is based on unsharp mask filtering (lungs adjusted to an optical density of 1.8, a gamma of 2.6, detail contrast enhancement of 0.4, and noise reduction of 0.8). The image matrix was 2 941 × 3 021 pixels, with a pixel size of 0.143 mm.

第 93 天

学习

According to the manufacturer's specifications, the exposure settings of the flat-panel detector radiography system used in this study were adjusted to provide a radiation dose equivalent to that of a 400-speed film-screen system. We assumed this would result in a dose reduction of approximately 50% compared with the conventional film-screen radiographs obtained with 200-speed film. Dose measurements were performed with a dosimeter using an anthropomorphic chest-phantom before the patient examinations, which were performed under identical exposure conditions (automatic exposure control using the same peak kilovoltage, tube current, grid, etc.) as for the patient examinations.

根据厂商的说明，此研究中所使用的平板探测器 X 线摄影系统的曝光装置，所应用的放射剂量已调整到等同于 400 速度屏 - 片系统所应用的放射剂量。我们估计这将导致 X 线剂量与 200 速度胶片所获得的传统屏 - 片 X 线照片相比大约降低 50%。在患者检查前用仿真胸部体模采用剂量仪进行剂量测试，这些是在相同曝光条件下进行的（采用相同峰电压、管电流、滤线栅等自动曝光控制）。

dosimeter [dəu'simitə] *n.* 剂量仪　　peak kilovoltage 峰电压

tube current 管电流

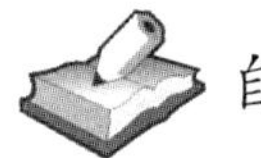

自测

我院螺旋 CT 由西门子 Somatom Plus 或 Plus-S 扫描机完成。用 2 mm 准直，床面行进速度 2 mm/s（螺距为 1）、210 mA、120 kVp。此技术使腕部的整个厚度在 20 ~ 24 s 能被成像。每隔 1 mm，用 180° 线性内插，并分别用软组织（410/7）、骨（2276/276）窗位照片进行兴趣区靶域的轴位重建。

答案

In our institution, helical CT is performed with a Siemens Somatom Plus or Plus-S Scanner with the spiral CT option. A 2-mm collimation is used with a table increment speed of 2 mm/s(pitch of 1) at 210 mA and 120 kVp. The entire thickness of the wrist can be imaged in 20—24 sec using this technique. Axial reconstructions of the targeted area of interest are performed every 1mm using 180° linear interpolation and are filmed using both soft-tissue (410/7) and bone (2276/276) window settings.

option ['ɔpʃən] *n.* 选择　　increment ['inkrəmənt] *n.* 增量、递增

soft-tissue window 软组织窗　　180° linear interpolation 180° 线性内插

bone window 骨窗

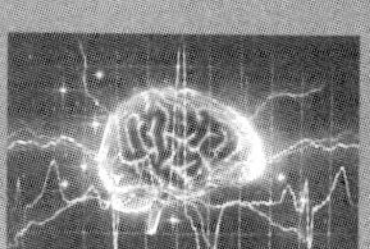

第 94 天

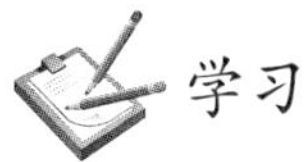
学习

For coronary CT angiography, collimation was 32mm × 0.6mm; section acquisition was 64 mm × 0.6 mm with the Z-flying focal spot technique; gantry rotation time was 330 ms; pitch was 0.20—0.43, adapted to heart rate; tube voltage was 120 kV; and maximum tube current was 400 mAs per rotation. For dose reduction, prospective tube current modulation was applied. Thereby, at heart rates less than 60 beats per minute, full tube current was applied from 60% to 70% of the cardiac cycle; at heart rates 60—70 beats per minute, from 50% to 80% of the cardiac cycle; and at heart rates higher than 70 beats per minute, from 30% to 80% of the cardiac cycle.

在冠状动脉 CT 血管成像中，准直器是 32 mm × 0.6 mm；获得层厚 64 mm × 0.6 mm，使用 Z 轴飞焦点技术；机架旋转时间 330 ms；螺距 0.20 ～ 0.43，适于心率；管电压 120 kV；最大管电流是 400 mAs/r。为降低剂量，利用管电流自动调节。所以，当心率＜ 60/min 时，心动周期的 60% ～ 70% 使用最大管电流；当心率为 60 ～ 70/min 时，心脏周期为 50% ～ 80%；当心率＞ 70/min 时，心脏周期为 30% ～ 80%。

fly focal spot technique 飞焦点技术

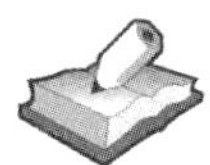
自测

对于数据重建，采用单扇区重建算法，图像重建采用两排探测器旋转 1/4 的数据。对于钙化积分，标准重建窗设置在 60% R-R 间期，采用非重叠影像：3 mm 有效层厚和中等锐利的卷积内核（B35f）。假如出现心律失常，R 波显示器将被手动调试来改善图像的同步质量。有效层厚是 0.75 mm，其重建增值是 0.4 mm。数据确定是通过使用中度软组织卷积核来滤过校准的（B26f）。

答案

For data reconstruction, a single-segment reconstruction algorithm was applied, which used the data of a quarter rotation of both detectors for image reconstruction. For calcium scoring, the standard reconstruction window was set at 60% of the R-R interval by using nonoverlapping images with 3 mm effective section thickness and a medium-sharp convolution kernel (B35f). In case of arrhythmia, R-wave indicators were manually adapted to improve the quality of synchronization. Effective section thickness was 0.75 mm, with a reconstruction increment of 0.4 mm. Data sets were filtered with a medium-soft convolution kernel (B26f).

score [skɔ:] *n.* 分数　　R-wave　R 波

synchronization [siŋkrənai'zeiʃən] *n.* 同步、使时间一致

reconstruction increment 重建增量　　convolution [kɔnvə'lu:ʃən] *n.* 卷积

single-segment reconstruction algorithm 单扇区重建算法

effective section thickness 有效层厚

第 95 天

学习

We performed a simple experiment to clearly illustrate the selenium memory artifact and to demonstrate that a single artifact can appear in multiple radiographic images. An X-shaped object was constructed of lead with approximate 4 mm thickness, and was radiographed at an exposure level frequently used in lateral chest examinations with the selenium system (150 kVp, 5 mAs). Immediately after the exposure, the lead X was removed and replaced with an anthropomorphic chest phantom. Two radiographic images of the chest phantom were acquired at 1 minute intervals after exposure of the lead X, with the use of routine imaging protocols (phototimed exposures at 150 kVp; at 1.8 and 1.9 mAs, respectively).

我们用以下的简单实验清晰地显示了硒记忆伪影的存在，并证明单个伪影能显示在多张X线摄影影像中。制作一个X形的铅箔，约 4 mm 厚，用硒系统对其进行拍摄，射线强度为侧位胸部检查时使用的强度（150 kVp、5 mAs）。曝光后即刻移去铅箔，换上类人胸部体模。在 X 形铅箔曝光后拍摄 2 张胸部体模的X线摄影影像，时间间隔为 1 min，使用常规拍摄（曝光条件为 150 kVp，分别用 1.8 mAs 和 1.9 mAs）。

自测

所有扫描在西门子 Somatom Plus 4 扫描机上获取，在 1.0 spr 扫描中（292 mA）用 120 kVp、292 mAs，在 0.75 spr 扫描中（也是 292 mA）用 219 mAs。完成所有扫描用 8 mm 准直器以及每旋转 1 周床速 8 mm（螺距为 1）。用 2 个连续螺旋扫描完整的腹和盆腔。以 3 ml/s 快速注射对比剂后 70 s 开始扫描。所有患者口服对比剂约 900 ml。所有扫描用相同的 180° 线性内插算法重建。

答案

All scans were obtained on a Siemens Somatom Plus 4 scanner at 120 kVp and 292 mAs for 1.0-spr scanning (292 mA) and 219 mAs for 0.75-spr scanning (also 292 mA). All scans were performed with 8mm collimation and a table speed of 8mm per rotation (pitch = 1). Two sequential helical scans were used to scan the entire abdomen and pelvis. Scanning began 70 after the initiation of a 3 ml/s monophasic bolus of contrast material. All patients had received

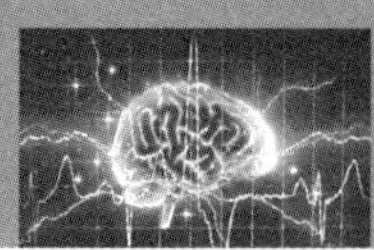

approximately 900ml of oral contrast material. All scans were reconstructed with the same 180° linear interpolation algorithm.

monophasic [mɔnə'feizik] *a.* 单相的　　bolus ['bəuləs] *n.* 团、块
oral contrast material 口服对比剂　　180° linear interpolation　180° 线性内插
initiation [iˌniʃi'eiʃən] *n.* 开始

第 96 天

学习

The examinations were performed with a phased array spine coil on a 1. 5 T imager equipped with a gradient-switching capability of maximally 25 mT/m in a rise time of 600 μsec. A single-shot turbo spin-echo sequence derived from the rapid acquisition with relaxation enhancement technique was used to obtain myelographic images. The parameters were effective TE, 850 ms; echo train length, 160; TR, 11.5 ms; matrix, 160 × 256; number of acquisitions, one; field of view, 125 mm × 200 mm; slice thickness, 20 mm; and acquisition time, 1.8 s. Because of the long TE, all background signals are suppressed except that from water. Coronal, sagittal, and left and right oblique views were obtained. All examinations were separately assessed at random by three observers.

在 1.5 T 影像机器上采用相控阵脊椎线圈完成检查，装备最大梯度场转换能力为在 600 μs 内改变 25 mT/m。从激励扫描与弛豫增强技术获得单次激发快速自旋回波序列，以获取脊髓影像。参数使用 TE 850 ms；回波链长度 160；TR 11.5 ms；矩阵 160 × 256；采集次数 1 次；视野 125 mm × 200 mm；层厚 20 mm；采集时间 1.8 s。因为 TE 时间长，除水以外所有背景信号被抑制。获取冠状、矢状和左、右倾斜影像。所有检查分别由 3 个观察者独立随机评价。

phased array coil 相控阵列线圈　　spine [spain] *n.* 棘、脊柱
gradient-switch 梯度开关
relaxation enhancement technique 弛豫增强技术
single-shot turbo spin-echo sequence 单次激发快速自旋回波序列
be derived from 从……产生的　　echo train length 回波链长度
slice thickness 层厚　　acquisition time 采集时间
coronal [kə'rəunəl] *a.* 冠状的　　sagittal ['sædʒitl] *a.* 矢状的
at random 任意、随机

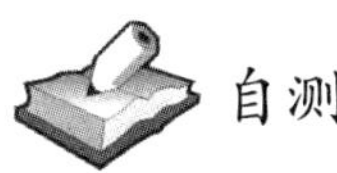

自测

活检线圈由一个引导装置和一个圆形表面线圈所组成。引导装置是一个直径为

4.5 cm 的圆柱形丙烯酸容器，稳固地套在表面线圈内。容器内填充了 0.5 mmol/L 的钆喷酸二甲基葡胺（Magnevist）溶液并具有 57 个穿刺管道（管径 1.2 mm），均与圆柱轴平行，且排列成 9 行。添加硝酸甘油胶囊于容器的顶部，以便认清病灶上方排列的管道。初步测试采用猪的组织标本表明，在容器和穿刺管道下方的组织标本能充分地显示含有 5 个模拟病变（即 5 mm 直径的 5 个硝酸甘油胶囊）。

The biopsy coil consists of a guiding device and a circular surface coil. The guiding device is a 4.5 cm-diameter cylindrical acrylic container that fits tightly into the opening of the surface coil. The container is filled with a 0.5 mmol/L solution of gadopentetate dimeglumine and has 57 puncture channels (1.2 mm lumen) that run parallel to the axis of the cylinder. The channels are arranged in nine rows. Nitroglycerol capsules affixed to the top of the container permit ready identification of the row situated directly above the lesion. Preliminary testing with a porcine tissue specimen showed that the container and the puncture channels were adequately depicted with respect to the underlying tissue sample, which contained five “lesions” (ie,5 mm-diameter nitroglycerol capsules).

puncture ['pʌŋktʃə] *n.* 小孔　　　surface coil 表面线圈
cylindrical [sə'lindrikl] *a.* 圆柱的、圆筒形的
acrylic [ə'krilik] *a.* 丙烯酸的、聚丙烯
gadopentetate dimeglumine [ˌgædə'pentəteit dgiˌmeglumiːn] 钆喷酸二甲基葡胺
capsule ['kæpsjuːl] *n.* 小盒、容器　　　porcine ['pɔːsain] *a.* 猪的
specimen ['spesimən] *n.* 标本、抽样

第 97 天

MR imaging in the breast was performed with a whole-body imager by using a dedicated bilateral breast surface coil. Among 170 consecutive patients, 157 underwent imaging with this compression device. In 13 patients, compression was not necessary because their breasts were large. The entire breast was imaged before and five times immediately after intravenous administration of gadopentetate dimeglumine, 0.1 mmol per kilogram of body weight. A two-dimensional fast low-angle shot, or FLASH, pulse sequence was used with a repetition time of 375 ms, an echo time of 5 ms, a flip angle of 90°, and an acquisition time of 87 seconds, which yielded thirty two 4 mm thick transverse sections without gaps. Postprocessing included subtraction of the unenhanced from the gadolinium-enhanced images on a pixel-by-pixel basis and presentation with the maximum-intensity-projection technique.

乳腺 MR 成像采用特定双侧乳腺表面线圈的全身成像仪完成。在连续的 170 例患者中，157 例采用这种压迫装置获得影像。13 例患者因乳腺大而无需压迫。静脉注射对比剂前、后立即获得 5 次整个乳腺成像，对比剂为钆喷酸葡胺每千克体重 0.1 mmol。采用二维快速小角度击发，或 FLASH 脉冲序列，重复时间 375 ms，回波时间 5 ms，翻转角 90°，采集时间 87 s，无间隔产生 32 个 4 mm 厚的横断面。后处理包括以一个像素对一个像素为基础的钆增强的影像与未增强的影像减影，并用最大密度投影技术显示。

whole-body imager 全身成像仪　　pulse sequence 脉冲序列
maximum-intensity-projection technique 最大密度投影技术
flip angle 翻转角

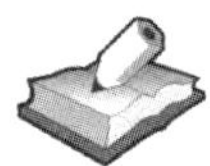

自测

下列的 MRI 序列用 1.0T 扫描仪获得：矢状位的重加权（TR/TE，3 800/16）和 T_2 加权（3 800/98）快速自旋回波（层厚 3 mm；扫描野 156 mm × 250 mm；矩阵 170 × 512），冠状位的 T_1 加权（608/20）自旋回波（层厚 4 mm；照射野 138 mm × 170 mm；矩阵 208 × 512），横断面的三维双回波稳态（30/9）梯度回波图像（层厚 2.7 mm；扫描野 140 mm × 140 mm；矩阵 256 × 256）和冠状位的 T_2 加权（4500/96）快速自旋回波脂肪抑制（层厚 4 mm；扫描野 135 mm × 180 mm；矩阵 210 × 512）。每个序列获取的时间为 2 min 18 s 到 4 min 35 s 不等。

答案

The following MR imaging sequences were acquired with the 1.0T scanner: sagittal intermediate-weighted (TR/TE, 3 800/16) and T_2-weighted (3 800/98) turbo spin-echo (section thickness, 3 mm; field of view, 156 mm × 250 mm; matrix, 170 × 512), coronal T_1-weighted (608/20) spin-echo (section thickness, 4 mm; radiation field, 138 mm × 170 mm; matrix, 208 × 512), transverse 3D double-echo steady-state (30/9) gradient-echo images (section thickness, 2.7 mm; field of view, 140 mm × 140 mm; matrix, 256 × 256), and coronal T_2-weighted (4 500/96) turbo spin-echo sequence with fat suppression (section thickness, 4 mm; field of view, 135 mm × 180 mm; matrix, 210 × 512). The acquisition times for each sequence varied between 2 min 18 s and 4 min 35 s.

turbo spin echo 快速自旋回波　　double-echo steady-state 双回波稳态
gradient echo 梯度回波　　fat suppression 脂肪抑制

第 98 天

学习

The MRI protocol on the 1.5T scanner included the following sequences: sagittal intermediate-weighted (3 760/14) and T_2-weighted (3 760/95) turbo spin-echo (section thickness, 3 mm; field of view, 143 mm × 180 mm; matrix, 204 × 512), coronal T_1-weighted (450/14) spin-echo (section thickness, 3 mm; field of view, 138 mm × 170 mm; matrix, 208 × 512), transverse 3D double-echo steady-state [multiecho data image (MEDIC)] (466/26) gradient-echo images (section thickness, 2 mm; field of view, 170 mm × 170 mm; matrix, 256 × 512), and coronal STIR (5 550/35; inversion time, 160 ms) (thickness, 3 mm; field of view, 135 mm × 170 mm; matrix, 203 × 512). The acquisition times for these sequences varied between 2 min 57sec and 4 min 38 s.

1.5T 扫描仪的 MRI 协定包含下列的序列：矢状位的重加权（3 760/14）和 T_2 加权（3 760/95）快速自旋回波（层厚 3 mm；扫描野 143 mm × 180 mm；矩阵 204 × 512），冠状位的 T_1 加权（450/14）自旋回波（层厚 3 mm；扫描野 138 mm × 170 mm；矩阵 208 × 512），横断面的三维双回波稳态［多回波数据图像 (MEDIC)］（466/26）梯度回波图像（层厚 2 mm；扫描野 170 mm × 170 mm；矩阵 256 × 512）和冠状位的 STIR（5 550/35；反转时间 160 ms）（层厚 3 mm；扫描野 135 mm × 170 mm；矩阵 203 × 512）。每个序列获取的时间在 2 min 57 s 到 4 min 38 s。

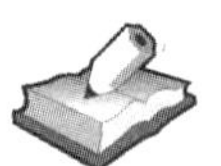

自测

影像在 5M 高分辨率黑白（灰阶）CRT 和 3M LCD 上显示。实际矩阵分辨率 LCD 是 2 048 × 1 536，CRT 为 2 560 × 2 048。LCD 理论上最大亮度是 515 堪德拉（candelas, cd/m^2），而 CRT 为 600 cd/m^2。CRT 荧光屏采用一个防反射罩。2 种显示器采用相同大小的屏（30 cm × 40 cm）。显示功能与基于 Barten 模型的 DICOM 标准一致，以确保在 2 种设备上影像显示稳定。2 种显示器最大亮度调至 300 cd/m^2；最小亮度尽可能低（≈ 0.3 cd/m^2）。进行判读时在周围同样亮度环境下制订最大亮度值和最小亮度值。

答案

Images were evaluated on a high-resolution 5-megapixel monochrome (gray-scale) CRT display and a 3-megapixel LCD. Actual matrix resolutions were 2 048 × 1 536 for the LCD and 2 560 × 2 048 for the CRT display. The theoretic maximum brightness was 515 candelas (cd)/m^2 for the LCD and 600 cd/m^2 for the CRT display. The CRT faceplate was covered by an antireflective coating. The two displays had equal screen sizes (30 cm × 40 cm). Display functions agreed with the DICOM standard based on the Barten model to ensure a consistent image appearance with both

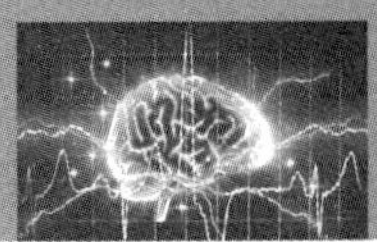

devices. Maximum luminance was adjusted to 300 cd/m^2 for both displays; minimum luminance was set as low as possible (≈ 0.3 cd/m^2). Maximum and minimum luminance values were set under the same ambient lighting conditions while the interpretation took place.

monochrome ['mɔnəkrəum] *n.* 黑白图像　　gray-scale 灰阶
candela [kæn'delə] *n.* 堪德拉（发光强度单位）
faceplate ['feispleit] *n.* 荧光屏　　antireflective *a.* 抗反射的

第 99 天

学习

Images were obtained with an automatic exposure control that was adjusted to provide a radiation dose equivalent to that provided by a 400-speed film-screen system. Exposure conditions were 125 kVp and 160 mA for the posteroanterior radiographs and 125 kVp and 250 mA for the lateral radiographs. The film focus distance was 180 cm. A grid (78 lines per centimeter; ratio, 13 : 1) was used. All digital images were processed with a standardized postprocessing set that was defined in collaboration with the manufacturer before the patient examinations. On the basis of the postprocessing algorithms supplied by the manufacturer, post-processing was adjusted to achieve a similar image appearance to the film-screen combinations used in our department. Briefly, the processing included a multiresolution algorithm to perform edge enhancement and dynamic range reduction and then applied an asymmetric sigmoidal look-up table to shape the contrast curve to match the screen-film combination. Finally, all digital images were transferred to a laser imager and printed on laser film.

用自动曝光控制放射剂量，使用相当于 400 速度屏 - 片系统所用的放射剂量来获取影像。对于后前位 X 线照片的曝光条件用 125 kVp 和 160 mA，侧位 X 线照片用 125 kVp 和 250 mA。焦 - 片距为 180 cm。使用滤线栅（78 lp/cm，栅比 13 : 1）。在患者检查前，所有数字图像都经与厂商双方认定的标准化后处理设备来处理。依据厂商提供的后处理算法，在我们科将后处理调整到与使用屏 - 片组合相似的影像显示。简单地说，处理包括使用多项分辨率算法来进行边缘增强和动态范围降低，然后应用非对称 S 形查找表使对比曲线平滑以匹配屏 - 片组合。最终，将所有数字影像传递给激光打印机并打印出激光照片。

automatic exposure control 自动曝光控制　　edge enhancement 边缘增强
dynamic range 动态范围
asymmetric [æsi'metrik] *a.* 不对称、不平衡
sigmoid ['sigmɔid] *n.* S 形；*a.* S 形的　　laser imager 激光相机
laser film 激光胶片

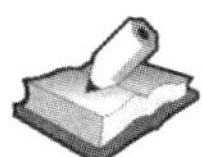

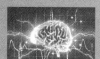

自测

多排探测器 CT 采用西门子 16 排探测器螺旋 CT 进行。患者进行扫描时保持正常心率,无抗心律失常药的应用(即, β - 受体阻滞药)。扫描参数为 120 kV、300 mAs,转速 420 ms, 16 mm × 0.75 mm 准直,每旋转 1 周床速 2.8 mm,平均扫描时间 23.4 s(范围 21.3 ~ 25.7 s), CT 剂量指数 41.96 mGy。扫描方向为头尾向扫描,从主肺动脉最尾端部分延长至膈。通过 18 号导管肘静脉注射,每个患者接受了 90 ml 非离子型对比剂。基于 Fleischmann 的研究,达到最优化增强方法进行主动脉 CT 血管造影: 30 ml 对比剂注射速度为 4.5 ml/s, 60 ml 对比剂注射速度为 2.5 ml/s, 30 ml 的氯化钠注射速度为 2.5 ml/s。使用注射触发技术,将 20 mm 直径兴趣区置于升主动脉,当注射对比剂的 CT 值达到 160 HU 时,开始自动触发扫描。

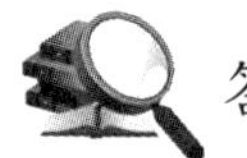

答案

Multi-detector row CT examinations were performed with a 16-detector row spiral CT scanner (Sensation 16; Siemens). Since the patients were scanned at their normal heart rate, no heart rate-controlling agents (ie, β -blockers) were used. Scanning parameters were 120 kV, 300 mAs, 420 ms gantry rotation speed, 16 mm × 0.75 mm collimation, 2.8 mm table feed per rotation, 23.4 s mean scanning time (range, 21.3—25.7 s), and 41.96 mGy CT dose index volume. The scanning direction was craniocaudal, and it extended from the most caudal parts of the main pulmonary artery to the diaphragm. Each patient received 90 ml of a nonionic contrast medium infused through an 18-gauge intravenous antecubital catheter. On the basis of the findings of Fleischmann, who researched optimal enhancement protocols for CT angiography of the aorta, a triphase protocol was applied for contrast medium administration: 30 ml of contrast material was administered at a rate of 4.5 ml/s, 60 ml of contrast material was administered at a rate of 2.5 ml/s, and 30 ml of sodium chloride was administered at a rate of 2.5 ml/s. With use of the bolus triggering technique , scanning was started automatically after contrast medium injection, as soon as an attenuation value of 160 HU was reached in a 20 mm-diameter region of interest placed in the ascending aorta.

agent ['eidʒənt] *n.* 剂
gantry rotation speed 机架旋转速度
CT dose index CT 剂量指数
main pulmonary artery 主肺动脉
diaphragm ['daiəfræm] *n.* 膈
antecubital [ˌænti'kjubitəl] *a.* 肘前的
aorta [ei'ɔ:tə] *n.* 主动脉;复数 aortae [ei'ɔ:ti:] 或 aortas
triphase ['traifeiz] *a.* 三相的
sodium chloride 氯化钠
bolus triggering technique 团注激发技术
diameter [dai'æmitə] *n.* 直径
region of interest 兴趣区
ascending aorta 升主动脉

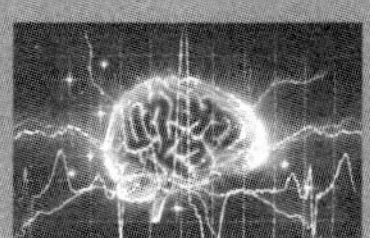

第100天

学习

Approximately 45 minutes before the start of image acquisition, patients received an intravenous injection of 300–400 MBq of FDG, which was produced in-house by using a 17.8 MeV cyclotron and an automated FDG synthesis module. All patients fasted for at least 4 hours before the examination. Just before scanning, the patients were asked to evacuate their bladders. First, two CT scans—one during normal expiration and one during maximum inspiration—were obtained from the pelvic floor to the head with the following parameters: 140 kV; 80 mA; 0.5 second per tube rotation; table speed, 38.5 mm/s; coverage, 867 mm; acquisition time, 22.5 seconds. Immediately after CT scanning, PET scanning was performed, again starting at the pelvic floor. This procedure is useful for minimizing the time between the acquisition of pelvic CT and PET images, which is necessary to minimize anatomic misregistrations caused by the filling of the bladder. Emission scans were obtained for 4 minutes per field of view and with one section overlap at the borders. Subsequently, PET transmission scans were obtained for 2 minutes per field of view.

大约在图像采集开始的前45 min要对患者静脉注射300 ~ 400 MBq的FDG。这些FDG是生产PET/CT系统的厂家机构内部生产的。生产这些FDG利用的是17.8 MeV的回旋加速器和自动的FDG化学合成模块。所有患者在检查前至少要禁食4 h。检查前，要求患者排空膀胱。首先，通过2种扫描方式对骨盆底到头部进行数据采集。这两种扫描方式是在平静呼气期间的扫描和在深吸气期间的扫描。扫描时的参数设置如下：140 kV、80 mA、球管每旋转1周0.5 s、诊视床移动速度38.5 mm/s、覆盖范围867 mm、采集时间22.5 s。CT扫描完成后，立即进行PET扫描。扫描范围仍从骨盆底部开始。减少CT扫描和PET扫描之间的时间间隔是很重要的，因为这必然会减少由于膀胱充盈引起解剖的错误显示是必要的。采用4 min/FOV放射扫描，并且使边界上的层面发生重叠。随后所进行的是2 min/FOV的PET透射扫描。

intravenous injection 静脉注射
cyclotron ['saikləutrɔn] *n.* 回旋加速器
synthesis ['sinθisis] *n.* 合成；复数 syntheses ['sinθisi:z]
module ['mɔdju:l] *n.* 模件
fast [fɑ:st] *vi.* 禁食
bladder ['blædə] *n.* 膀胱
evacuate [i'vækjueit] *vt.* 排空
inspiration [ˌinspə'reiʃən] *n.* 吸气
pelvic floor 盆底
table speed 床速
coverage ['kʌvəridʒ] *n.* 覆盖
misregistration 配准不良、位置不正
emission [i'miʃn] *n.* 发射
field of view 显示野（扫描野）
overlap [ˌəuvə'læp] *v.* 重叠
border ['bɔ:də] *n.* 边缘、边界
transmission [træns'miʃən] *n.* 透射

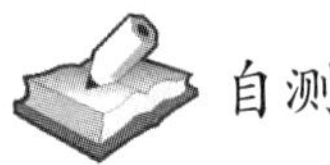
自测

采用心电回顾性门控技术对所有数据集图像重建,其特点是可以在心脏循环的任何阶段对数据集进行连续图像重建。重建参数为重建视野 220 mm,中度软组织核(B35 kernel),有效层厚 1.0 mm, 0.5 mm 增量。为影像评价采用窗宽 700 HU,窗位 100 HU。采用心脏重建算法为 16 排 CT(西门子)配备的标准心脏软件包进行图像重建。这种算法允许单扇区图像重建时心率低于 72/min,双扇区重建时心率高于 72/min。单扇区图像重建时间分辨率为 210 ms; 双扇区图像重建由于受心率影响,时间分辨率介于 105 ~ 210 ms。其中 210 ms 时间分辨率可应用于心率 72 ~ 96/min 的患者, 105 ms 时间分辨率可应用于心率 81 ~ 104 /min 的患者。在此心率范围之内,时间分辨率呈线性增加和减少。

答案

Image reconstruction in all data sets was performed by using retrospective electrocardiographic gating, a technique that allowed continuous image reconstruction from volume data sets during any phase of the cardiac cycle. Reconstruction parameters were 220 mm field of view, medium soft-tissue kernel (ie, B35 kernel), 1.0mm effective section thickness, and 0.5 mm increment. The window settings for image evaluation were window width of 700 HU and window level of 100 HU. The adaptive cardiac volume reconstruction algorithm, which is standardized and provided with the Sensation 16 (Siemens) cardiac software package, was used for image reconstruction. This algorithm allowed single-segment image reconstruction at heart rates slower than 72 beats per minute and two-segment reconstruction at heart rates faster than 72 beats per minute. With single-segment image reconstruction, temporal resolution was constantly 210ms; with two-segment image reconstruction, temporal resolution ranged from 105 to 210 ms, as influenced by the heart rate. A 210 ms temporal resolution was achieved at heart rates of 72 and 96 beats per minute, and a 105 ms temporal resolution was achieved at heart rates of 81 and 104 beats per minute. Between these heart rates, temporal resolution showed a linear increase and decrease.

retrospective electrocardiographic gate 回顾性心电门控
cardiac cycle 心脏周期
effective section thickness 有效层厚
increment ['inkrimənt] *n.* 增量
window width 窗宽
window level 窗位
reconstruction algorithm 重建算法
cardiac software package 心脏软件包
single-segment image reconstruction 单扇区影像重建
two-segment reconstruction 双扇区重建
temporal resolution 时间分辨率

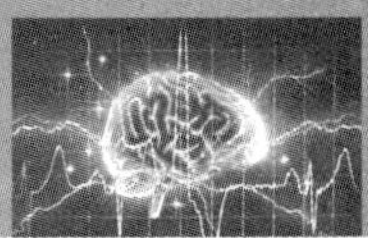

四、 评价方法

本节中作者须对其研究的内容采取何种评价方法进行说明，这里包括评判人，如评判人数、评判人的条件（资历）；分组，如何分组，分多少组，是否还有亚组；评判方法，如是否随机，是否采用盲法，评价方法是否齐同，如何设立参照组，以及如何打分等。

第 101 天

学习

Visual assessment of low-contrast resolution was performed by five experienced radiologists, who were blinded to the data acquisition system.

由 5 位有经验的放射学家对资料获得系统进行低对比分辨率显示的盲法评估。

The diagnoses that served as the reference standard were established by consensus of three radiologists who did not participate in the receiver operating characteristic (ROC) curve analysis. The consensus diagnoses were based on a review of CT scans and knowledge of each patient's history.

用作参照标准的诊断是由未参与 ROC 曲线分析的 3 个放射学家共同做出的。依据回顾每位患者的 CT 扫描及病史做出共同诊断。

consensus [kən'sensəs] *n.*（意见）一致，同意

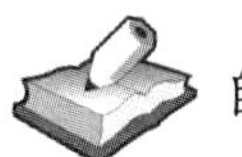

自测

对于数字及屏 - 片成像，观察者对各个影像有可能出现异常的评价采用 6 个等级表达，0 为确定正常，5 为确定异常。对临床诊断的结果可能无金标准（即没有绝对“正确”）。

允许观察者们随意观察 X 线片，如果需要可使用强光灯。没有时间或观片距离的限制。评价影像质量和确定包括肺实质、软组织和骨组织解剖结构的显示能力采用 5 分制进行评价（1 为不满意、2 为差、3 为一般、4 为好、5 为优秀）。

答案

For both digital and film-screen images, observers assessed each image with respect to the likelihood of abnormality using a six-point scale, with 0 being definitely normal and 5 being definitely abnormal. No gold standard was available with respect to clinical diagnosis (i.e., “truth” was not established).

gold standard 金标准

The observers were allowed to handle the films and to use a spotlight if desired. No time or viewing distance constraints were given. The image quality and the visibility of defined anatomic structures, consisting of lung parenchyma, soft tissue, and bone structures were evaluated using a 5-point scale (1 = unsatisfactory, 2 = poor, 3 = fair, 4 = good, 5 = excellent).

parenchyma [pə'reŋkimə] *n.* 实质　　　spotlight ['spɔtlait] 聚光灯

第 102 天

学习

Each radiologist subjectively analyzed image quality independently by visual assessment and rated the quality on a 4-point scale: 1. excellent (no limitations); 2. good (minor limitations, full diagnostic information); 3. moderate (major limitations, limited diagnostic information); and 4.poor visualization (nondiagnostic). Intermediate scores at 0.5 intervals were allowed.

各位放射学家通过视觉评估独立主观分析影像质量，在 4 个等级上判断质量：1. 优秀（无缺陷）；2. 好（较小缺陷，不影响整个诊断信息）；3. 适中（较大缺陷，影响诊断信息）；4. 显示差（不能诊断）。中间分数可间隔 0.5 分。

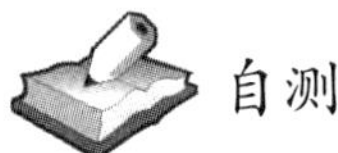

自测

2 种显示器并排放在同一平面上，以使光线对 2 种显示器都一样。房间内周围光线柔和（< 20lux）。显示器的显示不采用额外的影像处理。不进行在线处理，如放大及窗口技术。可根据个人喜好调节显示距离；对于 2 种显示器显示角接近 90°，以消除斜角显示效应。

答案

The two monitors were side by side on a standard table so that lighting conditions were identical for both. The ambient lighting in the room was subdued (< 20 lux). No additional image processing was applied for the monitor displays. No online processing, such as magnification or windowing, was available. Viewing distance could be adjusted to individual preference; viewing angle was consistently close to 90° with both displays to eliminate the effects of off-angle viewing.

monitor ['mɔnitə] *n.* 显示器　　　ambient ['æmbiənt] *a.* 周围的、环境的

subdue [səb'dju:] *vt.* 减弱、使光线柔和

magnification [ˌmægnifi'keiʃn] *n.* 放大、放大率、放大倍数

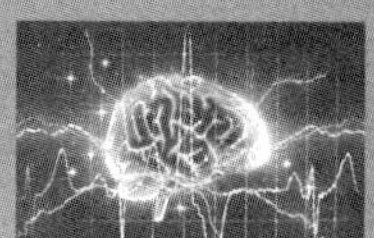

第 103 天

学习

Artifacts in the skin plane were evaluated in the maximum-intensity-projection images, and those within the parenchyma were evaluated in the subtraction images. A subjective classification was used: severe, moderate, or no artifacts. Severe artifacts were strong black and white lines that reduced the diagnostic value. Moderate artifacts were defined as fine lines that did not disturb the diagnostic value. No artifacts were defined as the appearance on images with optimal image subtraction.

在最大密度投影影像中评价皮肤表面的伪影，在减影影像中评价实质内的伪影。应用了一种主观分类：严重伪影、中等伪影或无伪影。严重伪影是粗的黑白线条以致降低诊断价值。中等伪影定义为细线条，不影响诊断价值。无伪影表现为最佳减影图像。

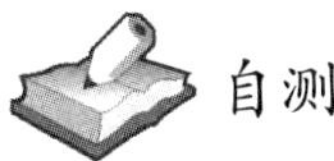
自测

图像评价由同样两个研究人员共同判读。为了避免研究人员偏差，评价图像质量和分析 CT 冠状动脉造影图像的时间间隔至少保持 4 周。所有数据随机进行评估，且重建间隔、重建技术和心率均为盲法评估。评估横断面图像、多平面重组技术（MPRs）、薄层最大密度投影技术（MIPs）。

答案

Image evaluation was performed by the same two observers in a consensus reading. To avoid observer bias, an interval of at least 4 weeks was kept between the evaluation of image quality and the analysis of CT coronary angiograms. All data sets were assessed in a random order and blinded with regard to the reconstruction interval, reconstruction technique, and heart rate. Transverse scans, MPR images, and thin-slab MIP images were assessed.

第 104 天

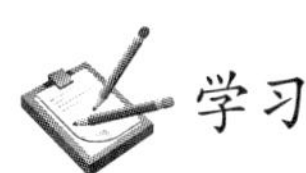
学习

The images were evaluated by seven radiologists, two of whom were senior chest radiologists, one with more than 15 years of experience in digital radiology. The other five were senior residents (fourth and fifth year). All radiologists were familiar with soft-copy interpretation of cross-sectional images on a CRT display but had variable experience with soft-copy interpretation of radiographic studies. All radiologists had only limited experience with LCD. Loading of images from the PACS workstation onto either monitor took less than 2 s. Evaluation time per image was unlimited.

由 7 位放射学家评价影像，其中 2 位是资深的胸部放射学家，其中 1 位具有 15 年以上数字 X 线摄影经验。其他 5 人为资深的住院医师（任职第 4 年或第 5 年）。所有放射学家熟悉在 CRT 显示屏上进行断面影像的软拷贝判读，但在 X 线照片软拷贝判读的研究中经验不一。他们对 LCD 经验有限。从 PACS 工作站下载影像到各个显示器小于 2 s。每幅图像的评价时间没有限制。

cross-sectional image 横断面影像　　cathode ray tube 阴极射线管，简称 CRT

liquid crystal display 液晶显示，简称 LCD

senior ['si:niə] *a.* 年长的、资历较深的

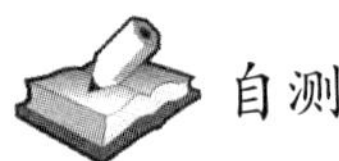 自测

观察者们评价各个影像采用 6 个等级表示影像质量，0 为非常差的影像质量，5 为优秀的影像质量。得出各个影像的全面质量的得分。此外，对于影像质量在 9 个不同的解剖部位上给予打分。这 9 个标记由下列每一个部位：腕骨、跗骨、胫骨、桡骨；掌骨、跖骨及指骨的软组织（脂肪界面及皮肤可见）、骨皮质（皮质边缘及滋养管可见）、骨小梁（各个骨小梁可见）组成。

 答案

Observers evaluated each image with respect to image quality using a six-point scale, with 0 being very poor image quality and 5 being excellent image quality. Each image was given an overall image quality score. In addition, each image was rated for image quality at nine specific anatomic locations (landmarks). These nine landmarks consisted of the soft tissues (visibility of fat planes and skin), cortical bone (visibility of cortical edges and vascular channels), and trabecular bone (visibility of individual trabecula) in each of the following locations:carpals, tarsals, tibia, and radius, metacarpals and metatarsals, and phalanges.

cortical ['kɔ:tikəl] *a.* 皮质　　trabecular [trə'bekjulə] *a.* 小梁

carpal ['kɑ:pl] *a.* 腕的　　tarsal ['tɑ:səl] *n.* 跗骨

tibia ['tibiə] *n.* 胫骨；复数 tibias 或 tibiae ['tibii:]

radius ['reidiəs] *n.* 桡骨；复数 radii ['reidiai]

metatarsal [ˌmetə'tɑ:sl] *n.* 跖骨

phalanx ['fælæŋks] *n.* 指骨、趾骨；复数 phalanges [fæ'lændʒi:z]

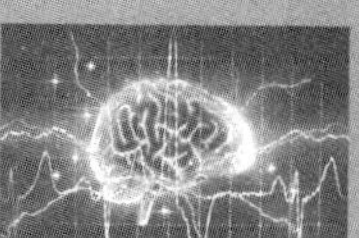

第 105 天

学习

【学习】

The conventionally attenuation-corrected PET images were used as references, and the other images were subjectively rated as having equal, acceptable, or lower quality. Image quality criteria were based on the anatomic position of organs adjacent to the diaphragm and the ^{18}F uptake in physiologic or pathologic structures. Thus, image quality was lower when, for example, the heart appeared anatomically displaced and the degree of FDG uptake in the myocardium appeared higher.

以常规衰减校正的 PET 图像作为参照，主观地评价其他图像：影像质量相当、影像质量可接受、影像质量差。图像质量的标准是基于与膈肌相邻的器官的解剖位置，以及生理或病理结构上对 ^{18}F 的摄取而定。因此，以心脏为例，当心脏在解剖上移位或者心肌对 FDG 的摄取显示较高时，图像的质量会降低。

organ ['ɔ:gən] *n.* 器官
uptake ['ʌpteik] *n.* 摄入、摄取
physiologic [ˌfiziə'lɔdʒik] *a.* 生理的、生理学的
pathologic [ˌpæθə'lɔdʒik] *a.* 病理的
myocardium [ˌmaiə'kɑ:diəm] *n.* 心肌

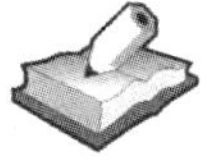
自测

CT 数据被传到一个离线工作站，由两个判读者评估，这两人对于有创冠状动脉造影和患者的临床信息不了解。诊断结果通过他们一致的阅片结果得出。评估 Agatston 的分数是采用半自动软件对非增强图像中 130 HU 以上部分进行评估。采用薄层最大密度投影、曲面重组和三维容量再现评估对比增强双源 CT。

答案

CT data were referred to an offline workstation and were interactively assessed by two readers who were blinded to the results of invasive coronary angiography and to clinical information. Decisions were reached with consensus reading. The Agatston score was assessed on unenhanced images with a detection threshold of 130 HU by using semiautomated software. Contrast-enhanced dual-source CT was evaluated by using thin-slab maximum intensity projection, along with curved planar reformation and three-dimensional volume rendering.

curved-planar reformation 曲面重组
volume render 容积再现

第 106 天

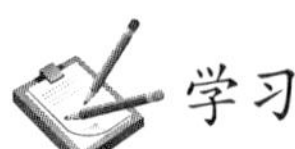
学习

The workstation was set up in an isolated room with constantly dimmed room lighting. The interpretation conditions closely simulated the clinical interpretation environment. For the soft-copy display, all images were loaded onto the hardware of the PACS workstation, on which it took less than 1 s for the observer to display any image. The software package in the workstation included such features as advance to the next case, real-time contrast and brightness adjustment, zoom via pixel replication, and contrast reversal. All digital operations were performed with a mouse.

工作站建立在一个孤立的房间内,其光线相对较暗。判读的条件与临床判读环境十分相似。软拷贝的显示影像载入 PACS 工作站的硬件上,观察者显示任何影像需时少于 1s。工作站的软件包括下述的先进性能:适时对比及亮度调节,通过像素复制的图像放大,以及对比反转。所有数字操作采用鼠标进行。

isolate ['aisəleit] *vt.* 隔绝

dim [dim] (dimmed; dimming) *v.* 变暗淡; dim out 遮暗

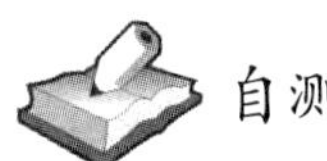
自测

采用下列计分系统评价诊断泌尿系结石: 1. 肯定阴性; 2. 可能阴性; 3. 不能判定; 4. 可能阳性; 5. 肯定阳性。其次,用解剖学的能见度来判断影像质量的好坏,采用下列计分系统评估: 1. 差; 2. 中等; 3. 优秀诊断。最后,分别记录各个部分所需的判读时间。记录这些应答并依据各自的系统进行统计学分析。

答案

The presence or absence of urinary calculi was evaluated using the following scoring system: 1. definitely negative; 2. probably negative; 3. indeterminate; 4. probably positive; and 5. definitely positive. Second, the image quality for interpretation, which focused on anatomic conspicuity, was evaluated using the following scoring system: 1. poor; 2. fair; and 3. excellent for diagnosing. Finally, the required time for interpretation in each session was recorded individually. These responses were recorded and resorted by each system for statistical analysis.

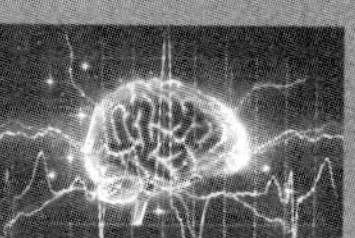

第 107 天

学习

Image quality was classified for each segment as being excellent (absence of artifacts related to motion or coronary calcification), as indicated with a score of 1; good (minor artifacts), score of 2; moderate (considerable artifacts but maintained visualization of arterial lumen), score of 3; or poor (nondiagnostic because of severe motion artifacts or extensive wall calcification), score of 4. Segments were visually scored for the presence of significant stenosis (≥ 50% narrowing in luminal diameter).

图像质量分类，优秀（无运动相关的伪影存在或冠状动脉钙化），被描述为 1 分；好的（较少伪影），为 2 分；中等的（相当多的伪影但可显示血管腔）为 3 分；或者差的（因为严重的移动伪影或者广泛的壁钙化而无诊断意义）为 4 分。对显著狭窄的部分进行打分（≥ 50% 的管腔狭窄）。

arterial [ɑ:'tiəriəl] *a.* 动脉的

lumen ['lu:men] *n.* 腔；复数 lumens 或 lumina ['lu:minə]

luminal ['lju:minəl] *a.* 腔的

stenosis [sti'nəusis] *n.* 狭窄；复数 stenoses [sti'nəusi:z]

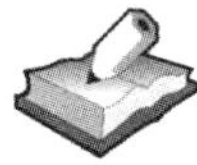

自测

11 位放射学家采用标准协定对这 3 套影像进行比较。其中有 3 位是资深的泌尿系放射学家，均有 20 年的工作经验，2 位为泌尿系成像方面专家。他们的临床实践是专门从事泌尿系成像。其他 8 位观察者是资深住院医师。所有观察者习惯于 PACS，因为他们在每天的实践中都在使用它。随机分发的这 3 套 X 线照片，分 3 部分每隔 1 周进行判读。各个观察者不知道患者的病史，且独立判读每一幅影像。

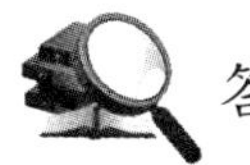

答案

Eleven radiologists compared these three sets of images using a standardized protocol. Three of the 11 observers were senior urologic radiologists, each with 20 years' experience, and two had fellowships in urologic imaging. Their clinical practices involved urologic imaging almost exclusively. The other eight observers were senior residents. All observers were accustomed to PACS because they used it in their daily practice. Interpretations of three sets of randomly distributed radiographs were performed individually in three separate sessions held at 1-week intervals. Each observer was unaware of the patient's history and interpreted each image independently.

urologic [juərəu'lɔdʒik] *a.* 泌尿科的

第 108 天

学习

Hard-copy images were interpreted independently by three observers (a board-certified general radiologist and two residents in the sixth and second years of training). All observers had training in thoracic radiology. As described previously, the postprocessing of the digital radiographs was optimized to achieve a similar image appearance to the conventional radiographs. However, the images of both modalities were easy to distinguish because of the different film material and format. Images from the two modalities were analyzed separately to exclude a potential bias from the direct intermodality comparison. Patient names were either removed or obscured, and no information about patient history was given. Furthermore, all cases were presented in a randomized order.

由 3 位观察者（1 位高级职称的放射学专家、2 位分别有 6 年和 2 年训练的住院医师）独立判读硬拷贝影像。所有观察者在胸部 X 线摄影方面有过培训。如先前的描述，数字 X 线照片的后处理达到与传统 X 线照片影像相同的满意度。然而，由于胶片材料和格式的不同，两种方式的影像还是容易区分的。这两种方式的影像分别进行分析，以除去由于这两种方式之间的比较而产生的潜在偏差。去除或隐藏患者的名字，不提供病史信息。而且，所有病例均随机显示。

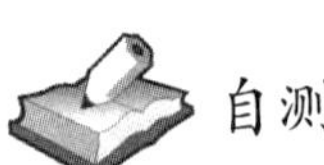

自测

模拟和数字影像由 4 位放射学家判读，他们在乳腺 X 线照片判读方面至少有 4 年临床经验。为了避免判读顺序影响，数字和传统影像的判读在不同时间进行。每套影像的显示顺序也不同。在判读数字影像前，给各位观察者在使用影像处理步骤方面作一个简单的介绍和实践时间。在观察模拟和数字乳腺 X 线摄影照片时，观察者们可自行调节最佳显示条件。他们必须根据 5 个参考等级给影像打分：1. 肯定不存在异常；2. 可能不存在异常；3. 不确定；4. 可能存在异常；5. 肯定存在异常。如果怀疑在数字影像上存在异常，观察者也必须在打分单上记录病灶的坐标。

答案

The analogue and digital images were read by four radiologists, each with at least 4 years of clinical experience in mammography. To avoid reading order effect, the digital and conventional images were interpreted on different days. The sequences of image presentation were also different for each set of images. Each observer was allowed a brief introduction and practice time on the usage of the image processing program before they interpreted the digital images. In

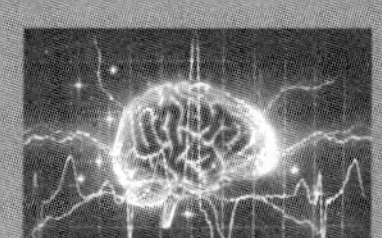

viewing the analogue and digital mammographic images, the observers were free to adjust their optimal viewing conditions. They had to score the images according to a five-point confidence scale: 1. abnormality definitely not present; 2. abnormality probably not present; 3. indeterminate; 4. abnormality probably present; 5. abnormality definitely present. If an abnormality on a digital image was suspected, the observer also had to record the coordinates of the lesion on the scoring sheet.

第 109 天

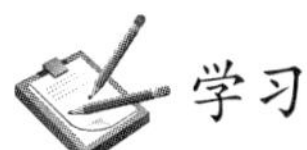

学习

Three general radiologists experienced in digital radiography were invited to evaluate a total of 200 images. The radiographs were presented to the independent radiologists in a random order on a computer workstation. Luminance of the screen was 260 cd/m2, the matrix was 1 000 × 1 000, and the diameter was 52 cm. Changes of window and density were allowed. Presentation of the full detector matrix was provided by a zoom function. The radiologists were unaware of any information related to the applied radiation dosage or patient history. The following anatomic regions and imaging features were evaluated: unobscured lung (not obscured by heart shadow or diaphragm); obscured lung (partially obscured by heart shadow or diaphragm); airways (trachea and main bronchi); mediastinum and pulmonary hilum; chest wall and bony thorax; and overall impression.

邀请 3 位在数字 X 线摄影方面有经验的放射学家评价所有的 200 份影像。在计算机工作站上这些图像被随机调出给各个放射学家。屏的亮度是 260 cd/m2，矩阵为 1 000 × 1 000，直径为 52 cm。允许进行窗和密度的调整。所有探测器矩阵的显示可通过图像放大功能进行放大。放射学家不知道任何与所用的放射剂量或病史有关的信息。根据下面解剖区域和成像特性进行评价：肺部清晰（心影或横膈没有模糊）、肺部模糊（心影或横膈部分模糊）、气道（气管和主支气管）、纵隔和肺门、胸壁和胸廓以及整体印象。

diaphragm ['daiəfræm] 膈，隔膜　　zoom [zu:m] *n.* 图像电子放大

trachea ['treikiə,trə'ki(:)ə] *n.* 气管；复数 tracheas 或 tracheae ['treikii:　trə'ki:i:]

dosage ['dəusidʒ] *n.* 剂量

bronchus ['brɔŋkəs] *n.* 支气管；复数 bronchi ['brɔŋkɑi]

mediastinum [ˌmi:diæs'tainəm] *n.* 纵隔；复数 mediastina [ˌmi:diæs'tainə]

pulmonary ['pʌlmənəri] *a.* 肺的　　hilum ['hailəm] *n.* 门

thorax ['θɔ:ræks] *n.* 胸，胸廓；复数 thoraxes 或 thoraces ['θɔ:rəsi:z]

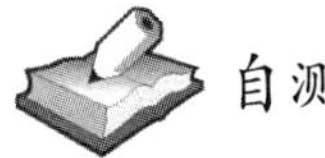

自测

5 位有经验的放射学家独立评判 50 只手或足的影像。观察者中的 4 位在肌肉骨骼放射

方面接受过专门的训练，1 位观察者刚刚经历放射科的实习期。影像采用随机法，以便先予以评价屏 - 片成像的一半，之后再评判它们相应的硒数字 X 线影像，反之亦然。一次性完成全部整套 50 幅影像的评价。首先评判一幅试验性影像。研究结果没有包括这些试验性成像的结果。采用相同的观片条件观察这些影像。这些条件由一个传统 X 线照片观片灯、一个热光源、一个放大镜，以及一个较暗的阅片室组成。

答案

Fifty foot or hand images were evaluated individually by five experienced radiologists. Four of them had subspecialty training in musculoskeletal radiology and one observer had just completed a radiology residency. Images were randomized so that one half of the film-screen images were evaluated before their selenium-based digital radiography counterparts, and vice versa. The complete set of 50 images was evaluated in one sitting. One practice image pair was evaluated first. The results of these practice images were not included in the results of the study. The images were observed using identical viewing conditions. These conditions consisted of a conventional radiography viewbox, a hot light, a magnifying glass, and a dimly lit reading room.

subspecialty [sʌb'speʃəlti] *n.* 亚专科

vice versa [ˌvaisi 'vəːsə] 反之亦然

residency *n.* 高级阶段

counterpart ['kauntəpɑːt] *n.* 一对中之一、副本

magnify ['mægnifai] *vt.* 放大

第 110 天

学习

In each of the 70 patients, the image quality of each eligible reconstruction interval (20 for relative timing and 20 for absolute timing; thus, 40 data sets per patient) was assessed separately by two independent observers who had at least 4 years of experience in interpretation of coronary CT angiograms. Each observer separately evaluated the images obtained in each of the 70 patients in a random order. The 40 data sets of each patient were evaluated by loading three-dimensional volume per three-dimensional volume. All data sets were blinded with regard to the reconstruction interval, reconstruction technique, and heart rate, and they were assessed in a random order. Image evaluation was performed on a separate workstation with a 512 × 512 image matrix and with use of thin-slab maximum intensity projection (MIP), multiplanar reformation (MPR), and transverse images. MPR and MIP were needed to determine the continuity of the vessel and the presence or absence of stair stepping; transverse images were needed to monitor in-plane movement.

由 2 位至少有 4 年判读 CT 冠状动脉图像经验的研究人员独立地对 70 例符合每个重

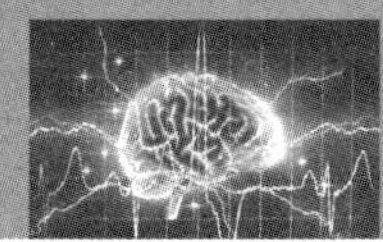

建间隔的患者图像进行质量评估（每例患者共 40 幅，相对时间 20 幅和绝对时间 20 幅）。每位研究人员分别随机评价这 70 例患者的图像。用三维体积来对每一个患者的 40 幅图像进行三维评价。对数据重建间隔、重建技术、心率等参数采用盲法评判，按随机次序来评估。图像评价由一个单独的工作站来处理，它的基本设置为 512 × 512 矩阵，配备常用的薄层最大密度投影技术（maximum intensity projection, MIP），多平面重组技术（multiplanar reformation, MPR），以及横断面影像。MPR 和 MIP 用来确定血管的连续性以及是否步进缺失；横断面成像用来监测平面运动。

reconstruction interval 重建间隔

maximum intensity projection 最大密度投影，简称 MIP

multiplanar reformation 多平面重组，简称 MPR

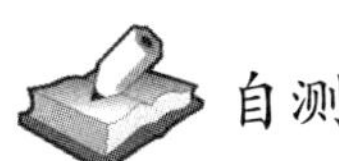

自测

图像质量评价分为 4 级：第 1 级优质图像质量；第 2 级良好的图像质量；第 3 级中等图像质量；第 4 级差的图像质量。优质图像质量表现为血管呈现连续过程，无阶梯伪影，在 MPR 图像或者 MIP 图像和横断面 CT 扫描时出现明亮的圆形或椭圆形，无运动伪影和四周低衰减的脂肪组织。良好的图像质量表现为在任何平面方向血管边缘可存在离散模糊，轻微的运动伪影 - 离散尾部或在横断面图像上的条纹伪影，在 MPR 图像或者 MIP 图像并没有阶梯伪影。中度的图像质量表现为血管明显模糊或离血管中心的运动伪影长度＜ 5mm，阶梯伪影小于血管直径的 25%。较差的图像质量表现为血管及其周围组织分界不清，离血管中心的条纹伪影长度至少 5mm，阶梯伪影超过血管直径的 25%。

答案

A four-step grading scale allowed classification into four groups: group 1, excellent image quality; group 2, good image quality; group 3, moderate image quality; and group 4, poor image quality. Excellent image quality was attributed to vessels showing a continuous course, without stair-step artifacts, appearing as bright circular or oval areas on MPR images or MIP images and transverse CT scans, without motion artifacts and surrounding low-attenuation fat tissue. Good image quality was classified as the presence of discrete blurring of vessel margin in any planar orientation, minor motion artifacts-seen as discrete tail or streak-emitting shadows on transverse images, and no stair-step artifact on MPR images or MIP images. Moderate image quality was classified as noticeably blurred vessels or plaque margins, distinctly broader motion artifacts extending less than 5mm from the vascular center, and stair-step artifact of less than 25% of the vascular diameter. Poor image quality was defined as an inadequate delineation between the vessels and surrounding tissues, the presence of streak artifacts extending at least 5mm from the center of the vessels, and stair-step artifacts of more than 25% of the vascular diameter.

classification [ˌklæsifi'keiʃən] *n.* 分类

moderate ['mɔdərit] *a.* 中等的、适度的

stair-step artifacts 阶梯伪影

circular ['səːkjulə] *a.* 圆形的、环状的、循环的

oval ['əuvəl] *a.* 卵圆的、卵形的

discrete [dis'kriːt] *a.* 分离的、分散的、稀疏的

blur [bləː] *v.* 变模糊

vessel ['vesl] *n.* 管、脉管

streak-emitting shadows 条纹放射影

plaque [plɑːk] *n.* 斑块

vascular ['væskjulə] *a.* 血管的、脉管的

第 111 天

学习

The digital data were also sent to a PACS server and distributed to display workstations. All images were down-loaded onto the local hard disk drives of the display workstations before being viewed by a radiologist. We used two viewer systems for soft-copy display: a high-resolution video monitor with 2 000 × 2 500 × 8 bit pixels used in a darkened room for side-by-side image display, and a liquid-crystal-display (LCD) monitor with 1 280 × 1 024 × 8 bits pixels. The monitors operated at 71 Hz in an interlaced mode and had a maximum brightness level of 100 foot-lamberts. The gray scale of digital images was modified by means of 10-to 8bit (storage phosphor image) look-up table. To eliminate the differences between the two monitors, their maximal brightness was adjusted to be the same. The soft-copy images were displayed without unsharp masking. Only window width and image level were automatically optimized by the customized program. The observers were allowed to adjust the brightness and contrast of the images. Localized magnification of each image was also permitted. For this observer performance study, patient identification was obscured on all images and was replaced by a sequence number.

数字资料也发送到 PACS 服务器并送给显示工作站。在放射学家观看之前所有影像下载到本机工作站显示的硬盘驱动器上。我们采用两套观察系统用于软拷贝的显示：一个是具有 2 000 × 2 500 × 8 bit 像素在暗房内并列显示影像的高分辨率图像显示器，一个是具有 1 280 × 1 024 × 8bit 像素的液晶显示器。显示器在 71 Hz 间隔上运行，且最大亮度为 100 英尺朗伯（foot-lamberts，亮度单位）。以 8 ～ 10 bit（荧光存储影像）检查表修改数字影像的灰阶。为了消除 2 台显示器间的差异，将它们的最大亮度调制到一样。软拷贝影像不用非锐化屏蔽显示。只有窗宽和窗位由程序自动优选。观察者可以调制影像的亮度与对比度。也允许各个影像的局部放大。为了观察者进行这种研究，所有影像上消除患者信息并以系列数字来代替。

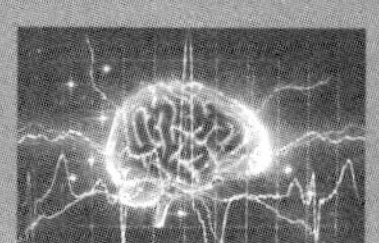

lambert ['læmbə:t] *n.* 朗伯（亮度单位，物体表面垂直方向上每平方厘米反射或辐射一“流明”的亮度）

foot-lambert 英尺朗伯（亮度单位）　　interlace [intə'leis] *n.* 间隔

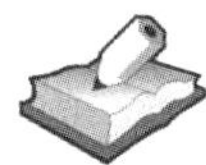

自测

3 位有骨骼肌 MRI 经验并应用 PACS 的读片者对检查进行评价。读片者 1 是一位专门从事骨骼肌放射，包括使用 MRI 有 5 年工作经验，并有例行从事用于此研究的 PACS 1 年经验的放射科住院医师。读片者 2 是位骨骼肌 X 线工作者及具有 MRI 1 年的工作经验，包括 4 个月的骨骼肌 MRI 的特别培训和 4 个月这项研究中应用 PACS 的经验。读片者 3 是位有着 5 年的膝关节 MRI 的实践经验和 1 年应用 PACS 经验的初级整形外科医师（虽然他习惯于基于网络的 PACS 观察，但屏幕设计和图像触摸特征与这项研究中以工作站为基础的不一样）。3 位评审员都知道患者都已经在 MRI 以后接受了关节镜检查或者外科手术。然而，他们对 MRI 诊断和临床、手术发现一无所知。为了减少认识和学习的偏差，图像分析（硬拷贝和软拷贝）的顺序分别在第 20、40 和 60 位患者以后发生改变。20 人一组的检查硬拷贝和软拷贝的评价至少间隔 1 周。

答案

Three reviewers with varying experience in musculoskeletal MRI and with the PACS evaluated the examinations. Reviewer 1 was a staff radiologist who had been specializing in musculoskeletal radiology, including MRI, for 5 years and who had routinely worked with the PACS used in this study for 1 year. Reviewer 2 was a fellow in musculoskeletal radiology with 1 year of experience in MRI, including 4 months of specific training in musculoskeletal MRI and 4 months of experience with the PACS used in this study. Reviewer 3 was a junior staff member in orthopedic surgery with 5 years of practical experience with MRI of the knee and 1 year of experience with PACS (although he was accustomed to the Web-based PACS viewer, the screen design and image handling features of which were in part different from the workstation-based version used in this study). The three reviewers were aware that patients had undergone arthroscopy or surgery after MRI. However, they were blinded with the prospective MRI diagnosis and the clinical and intraoperative findings. To reduce recognition and learning bias, the order of image interpretation (hard copy and soft copy) was changed after 20, 40, and 60 patients. The evaluation of soft copies and hard copies was at least 1 week apart within the groups of 20 examinations.

junior ['dʒu:njə] *n.* 年少者　　orthopedic [ˌɔ:θəu'pi:dik] *n.* 矫形外科学

prospective [prə'spektive] *a.* 预期的、未来的

recognition [rekəg'niʃən] *n.* 识别、认出

五、 统计分析

有了以上这些病例资料、影像设备、技术条件、评价方法之后，通过什么来确保其研究的正确性呢？这就需要依靠统计学对数据加以分析，对数据进行分门别类地处理。一句话，一篇文章的科学性就是通过统计学来反映的，没有统计学的文章，从严格意义的角度来讲就构不成一篇科研论文。反过来，也只有统计学才能保证一篇论文的科学性。然而，诸多的统计学方法都有其适用范围，这就需要选择恰当的统计学方法，合理地加以应用，只有这样才能确保其分析的科学性和正确性。

第 112 天

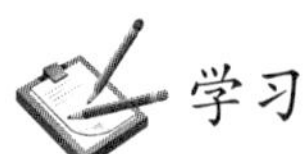

学习

A traditional paired *t* test was also performed to ascertain whether the average image quality of one technique could be considered statistically and significantly superior to the other.

本研究也做了传统配对 *t* 检验，以确定一种技术的平均影像质量是否被认为在统计学意义上优于另一种技术。

注：*t* test 适用于方差齐性与正态分布的定量统计，有样本均数与总体均数的比较、配对设计定量资料的比较、完全随机设计两样均数的比较。

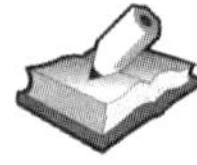

自测

以各个标准、各位放射学家及各种成像方式计算平均值。对于不同数字影像的最终得分，各组样本（95% 可信区间）采用双边配对样本 Student's *t* 检验进行比较。共分析了 3 600 次观测。

答案

Mean values were calculated for each criterion, each radiologist, and each imaging modality. The resulting values for the different digital images were compared by using two-tailed Student's *t* test for paired samples (confidence level, 95%). A total of 3 600 observations were analyzed.

confidence level 可信度

注：two-tailed Student's *t* test for paired samples 为两组样本的配对 *t* 检查。配对设计方法主要有：每对受试对象分别接受两种不同的处理；同一受试对象分别接受两种不同的处理。配对样本 *t* 检验使用的前提条件是：两个样本必须是配对的，这里面包括两个样本的观察值数目相同，两个样本观察值的顺序不随意更改；第二是样本来自两个总体，必须服从正

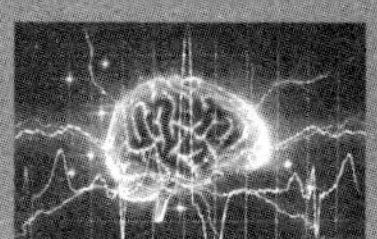

态分布。再根据方差是否齐性决定其使用的统计学方法。

第 113 天

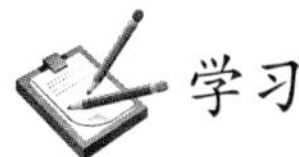

For the question of for which observers can the sum of image quality ratings for the nine landmarks be considered equivalent for digital and film-screen radiography, 90% confidence intervals were constructed for the true average difference between digital and film images in terms of the sum of the nine landmark image quality ratings. In addition, a traditional paired *t* test was performed to ascertain whether the average sum for one technique could be considered statistically and significantly higher than the other. This test was performed at the 0.05 significance level.

对于哪些观察者能对数字及屏 - 片 X 线摄影的 9 个标记点图像质量的总体评价被视为等同这一问题，90% 的可信区间构成真正平均差。此外，还做了传统配对 *t* 检验，以确定一种技术的平均总和是否在统计学上明显高于另一技术。这种检验在 0.05 显著水平下进行。

ascertain [æsə'tein] *vt.* 确定、查明

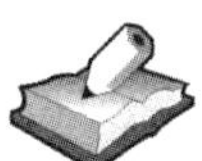

为了评价哪一个标记点及哪一个观察者对数字及屏 - 片 X 线影像质量的主观评判可被视为等同，采用 Obuchowski 的方法进行配对 *t* 检验。进行这些 *t* 检验显著水平定在 0.05。此外，在数字及屏 - 片影像间的主观评价影像质量方面，真实平均差确立为 90% 的可信区间。

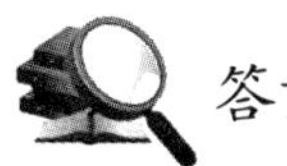

To evaluate for which landmarks and for which observers the subjective assessments of the image quality of digital and film-screen radiography could be considered equivalent, paired *t* tests were performed using the method suggested by Obuchowski. These tests were performed at a 0.05 level of significance. In addition, 90% confidence intervals were constructed for the true average difference in subjectively assessed image quality between digital and film-screen images.

第 114 天

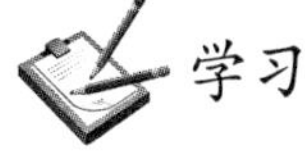

Results were expressed as means ± standard deviations. A linear mixed-effects model (SAS, version 9.1) was used to compare root-mean-square error between images. A *P* value of less than

0.05 was considered to indicate a significant difference.

结果被表示成平均值 ± 标准差。用一个线性的混合效应模型（9.1 版的 SAS）与图像间的均方根相比较。$P < 0.05$ 有显著差异。

statistical analysis software 统计分析软件，简称 SAS

root-mean-square 均方根

注：standard deviation 标准差，直接地、总结地、平均地描述了变量值的离散程度，在同质的前提下，标准差越大，这一组资料的变异程度越大。

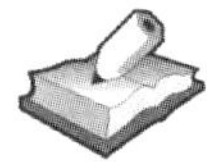 自测

用 Wilcoxon 检验和 Mann-Whitney 检验完成统计学评价。

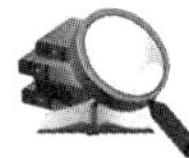 答案

Statistical evaluation was performed with the Wilcoxon test and the Mann-Whitney test.

注：Wilcoxon test 有 Wilcoxon signed-rank test 和 Wilcoxon rank sum test 两种，前者为配对设计差值比较的符号秩检验，适用于检验差值的总体中位数是否等于零；后者适用于完全随机设计的两个样本均数比较，不满足 t 检验条件的定量资料或等级资料。

Mann-Whitney test 两个独立样本的非参数检验，用于对两总体分布的比较判断。

第 115 天

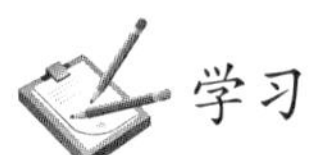 学习

Wilcoxon rank sum test was used to assess the significance of differences between ratings at a P level of less than 0.05. This was performed on a reviewer-by-reviewer basis and after averaging the scores over the seven radiologists.

用 Wilcoxon's 秩和检验评价 2 种率之间 $P \leqslant 0.05$ 差异的显著性。这是对每位评判者分别进行并计算 7 位放射学家的平均得分后得出的。

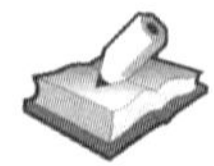 自测

我们对各种方式的影像质量和解剖结构都做了平均值和标准差的测定。采用 Wilcoxon 标记秩检验对数字 X 线摄影系统和屏 - 片 X 线摄影系统所获影像间的显著性差异做了测试。

 答案

Mean values and standard deviations were calculated for the image quality and anatomic

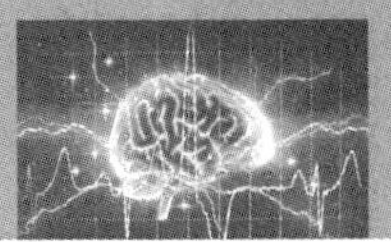

structures for each modality. Differences between the images obtained with the digital radiography system and the film-screen radiography system were tested for significance using the Wilcoxon's signed rank test.

注：mean value 均数，反映一组观察值的平均水平，适用于单峰对称或近似单峰对称分布资料的平均水平的描述。

Wilcoxon's signed rank test 又称 Wilcoxon 符号秩检验，用于非参数配对设计，以检验差值的总体中位数是否等于零。

第 116 天

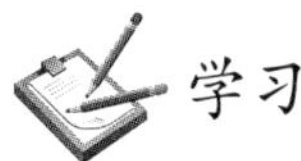

学习

The level of agreement between digital and film-screen radiography with respect to likelihood of abnormality was assessed through the use of the weighted kappa statistic (rather than the standard kappa statistic, because of the ordinal nature of the scale used) to measure the degree of agreement between digital and film-screen radiography. In addition, 95% confidence intervals for the true value of weighted kappa were calculated.

通过采用加权 *K* 检验评价（不用标准 *K* 检验，因为采用等级为自然序数的缘故）在数字与屏 - 片 X 线摄影之间关于可能出现异常情况的一致性从而测量数字与屏 - 片 X 线摄影的一致性。此外，计算了加权 *K* 真实值 95% 的可信区间。

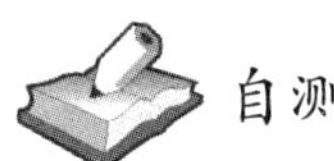

自测

可用 *K* 检验统计计算研究人员间对图像质量的认同。结果被解释为差（$K < 0.20$），一般（ K=0.21 ~ 0.40），中等（K=0.41 ~ 0.60），好（K=0.61 ~ 0.80），良好（K=0.81 ~ 0.90），或优秀（$K > 0.91$）。以标准方法计算得出 95% 可信区间（confidence interval, CI），$P < 0.05$ 表示统计学上存在明显的差异。

答案

Agreement between the investigators in the grading of image quality was calculated with the *K* statistic. Results were interpreted as poor ($K < 0.20$), fair (K = 0.21—0.40), moderate (K = 0.41—0.60), good (K = 0.61—0.80), very good (K = 0.81—0.90), or excellent ($K > 0.91$). A 95% confidence interval (CI) was calculated with a standard method and assigned to each value. A *P* value of less than 0.05 was considered to indicate a statistically significant difference.

P value　*P* 值　　　statistically significant difference 显著的统计学差异

第 117 天

Any influence of the heart rate on image quality was analyzed by using the Spearman correlation analysis. Correlation variables were the heart rate and the prevailing best image quality obtained at that heart rate. A *P* value of less than 0.05 was considered to indicate a statistically significant difference.

以 Spearman 相关分析分析心率对图像质量的影响。心率与对应心率获得的最佳图像质量之间呈现相关关系。$P < 0.05$ 表示统计学上存在明显的差异。

Spearman correlation analysis　Spearman 相关分析

prevail [pri'veil] *vi.* 占优势，经常发生

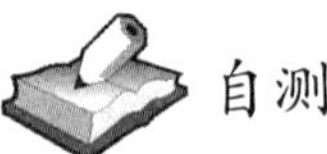

多排探测器 CT 冠状动脉造影及有创冠状动脉造影在冠状动脉粥样硬化相关性程度采用 Spearman 相关分析。多排探测器 CT 冠状动脉造影中出现的数据分布对称和高估或低估的数据将采用 Bowker 检验校正。

The degree of correlation between multi-detector row CT coronary angiography and invasive coronary angiography in grading of coronary atherosclerosis was investigated with Spearman correlation analysis. The symmetry of data distribution and any underestimation or overestimation with multi-detector row CT coronary angiography were checked with the Bowker test.

atherosclerosis *n.* 粥样硬化　　symmetry ['simitri] *n.* 对称

第 118 天

Because the image quality and visibility of the anatomic structures in this study were rated subjectively by the observers, an assessment of interobserver agreement was desirable to get an impression of the objectivity and reliability of the image evaluation. Kappa statistics were not applicable because of the large number of multivariate responses caused by the number of observers and response categories. Instead, Spearman's rank correlation was performed for all criteria for all observer combinations. The level of significance was calculated for each

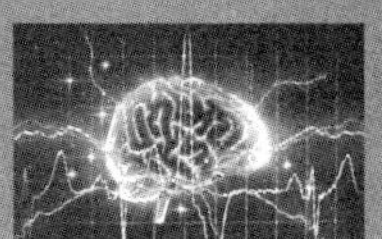

correlation.

因为在此研究中，解剖结构的影像质量和显示是依据观察者们的主观判断做出的，所以为了能得到影像评价的客观和可信印象，需要观察者一致的评估。由于观察者们和反应类别的数量导致大量多变量响应，所以 *K* 检验不能被应用。取而代之用 Spearman 的秩相关对所有观察者组合标准进行统计。对各个相关性进行显著性水平统计。

Spearman's rank correlation Spearman 秩相关，是用双变量等级数据做直线相关分析，适用于：不服从双变量正态分布而不宜做积差相关分析，总体分布型未知，原始数据是用等级表示。它是用秩相关系数 r_s 来说明两个变量间相关关系的密切程度与相关方向。

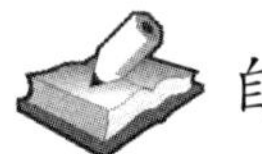

自测

Spearman 相关分析也被用来评估心率水平和在绝对与相对重组时间隔中 R-R 的起始点对最佳图像质量的可能影响。如无显著性差异，将用 McQueen-Rubin 聚类分析找出可能的群或亚群数据。两种分析分别应用于左右冠状动脉和冠状动脉左旋支的近段、中段和远段。如果聚类分析为阳性，用单变双聚无歧视分布分析来确定集群之间可能的截止心率。

答案

The Spearman correlation analysis was also used to evaluate a possible relationship between the level of the heart rate and the R-R starting points of the relative and absolute reconstruction intervals leading to best image quality. In case of nonsignificant results, McQueen-Rubin cluster analysis was used to enable identification of possible subgroups or "clusters" of data. Both analyses were performed separately for proximal, medial, and distal sections of the RCA, LCA, and LCX, respectively. In case of positive findings at cluster analysis, univariate two-population distribution-free discrimination analysis was used to determine possible cutoff heart rates between the clusters.

第 119 天

学习

Statistical analysis was performed with software (version 6, SAS). A *P* value of less than 0.05 indicated a statistically significant difference. Quantitative variables were expressed as means ± standard deviations; categoric variables were expressed as frequencies or percentages. Values of image quality are given in means ± standard deviations. Impact of heart rate, heart rate variability, or calcification on mean image quality per patient was tested by using multivariate linear regression analysis and effect testing. Thereby, heart rate was defined as mean heart rate during examination; heart rate variability refers to the maximal spread of heart rate during examination. Calcification is quantified by Agatston score.

统计学分析是通过软件 (version 6, SAS) 进行的。$P < 0.05$ 时具有显著统计学差异。定量差异表达：均值 ± 标准差；定性表达：频率或者百分数。图像质量是均值 ± 标准差。病人心率、心率化和钙化对图像平均质量的影响是通过使用多元线性回归分析来进行测定。因此，心率被定义为在测试过程中的平均心率；心率变化被定义为在测试过程中心率的最大波动。钙化可通过 Agatston 表来评判。

linear regression analysis 直线回归分析，是用直线方程来描述两个变量之间的线性关系。经典的线性回归要求资料满足：线性、独立性、正态性、方差齐性，其中 LINE 是经典线性回归的核心。

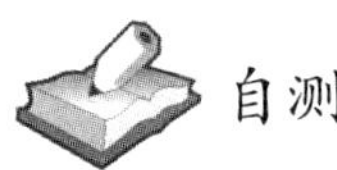
自测

对于 ROC 分析，由 4 位授权的不同放射学家采用相同的标准做进一步影像评价。要求放射学家采用下列 5 个可信度等级确认各个集体与单个标准是否可见：1. 确定不存在；2. 可能不存在；3. 不确定；4. 可能存在；5. 明确存在。此外，观察者在肺的图片上标出病变部位。分别有 80 幅数字和传统影像，且都具有后前位及侧位 X 线照片。为了避免判断上的偏差，把数字和传统影像随机地分发给各个观察者。这些观察者各自分别评价数字和传统 X 线检查。观看同一患者的检查要有时间间隔，至少 6 周以使记忆作用降至最低。观察者不回顾病史。在相同条件下进行影像评价，如房间光线及观片灯；判断时间无限制。

答案

For the ROC analysis, further image evaluation using the same list of criteria was performed independently by four different board-certified radiologists. The radiologists were asked to determine whether each collective and single criterion was visible using the following five-level rating scale of confidence:1. definitely not present; 2. probably not present; 3. equivocal; 4. probably present; 5. definitely present. In addition, the observers noted the location of the lesion on a diagram of the lung. There were 80 digital and 80 conventional image-pairs, each consisting of posteroanterior and lateral radiographs. Digital and conventional image-pairs were given to the observers in randomized order to avoid bias in interpretation. The observers had to evaluate the digital and conventional examinations separately. Examinations of the same patient were viewed with a time interval of at least 6 weeks to minimize learning effects. Observers were not aware of the patient's history. Image evaluation was always performed under equal conditions such as room light or viewing boxes; interpretation time was unlimited.

randomize ['rændəmaiz] *vt.* 使随机化　　bias ['baiəs] *n.* 偏见、倾向性、癖好

receiver operating characteristic 缩写为 ROC，受试者作业特征曲线。以计算曲线面积来

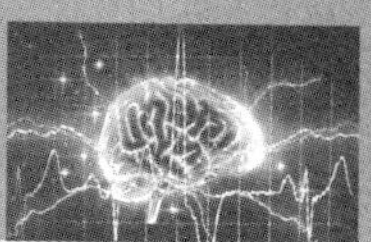

评价图像质量优劣，是主观的一种评价方法。

第 120 天

学习

To evaluate the observer's preference in detecting urinary calculi and the considered various viewing methods, the COR ROC2 program was used to calculate the receiver operating characteristic curve area and its standard deviation for a given observer's results. The average receiver operating characteristic areas from all observers using various visualization formats were compared using the paired Student's *t* test. The difference in image quality for each observer, according to the different viewing methods, was also compared using the paired *t* test ($P < 0.05$).

为评价观察者在诊断泌尿系结石中的选择并考虑不同的观察方法，利用 COR ROC2 程序计算受试者作业特征曲线（receiver operating characteristic curve, ROC 曲线）面积和各观察者结果的标准差。采用配对 *t* 检验来比较使用不同影像方式的所有观察者的平均 ROC 面积。同时采用配对 *t* 检验（$P < 0.05$），比较不同观察方法下每个观察者的影像质量差异。

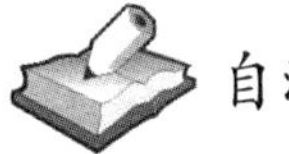
自测

根据 McNemar 检验来评价诊断性能（敏感性、特异性和准确性）中的差异。用 Bonferroni 检验中的方差分析评估诊断和评估时间中可信度差异的 hoc 比较。$P < 0.05$ 被认为有统计学意义。使用 kappa 统计来评估观察者间的一致性。根据 Landis 和 Koch，一致性评估如下：0 ~ 0.20 的 kappa 值表示轻度一致，0.21 ~ 0.40 表示一般一致，0.41 ~ 0.60 表示中等一致，0.61 ~ 0.80 表示较好的一致，超过 0.81 可认为是极好的一致。完全一致就是 1.00。我们采用 SPSS 软件 10.0 版本在 Windows（微软）环境下操作。

答案

Differences in diagnostic performances (sensitivity, specificity, and accuracy) were evaluated using the McNemar test. Differences in the confidence of the diagnosis and evaluation times were assessed with analysis of variance in the Bonferroni test for post hoc comparisons. Values for *P* of less than 0.05 were considered to be statistically significant. Interobserver agreement was assessed using kappa statistics. According to Landis and Koch, the agreement was rated as follows: a kappa value of 0—0.20 indicated slight agreement; 0.21—0.40 indicated fair agreement; 0.41—0.60, moderate agreement; 0.61—0.80, substantial agreement; and greater than 0.81, excellent agreement. Absolute agreement would be 1.00. We used SPSS for Windows (Microsoft) software, version 10.

McNemar test 一种变化显著性检验，它将研究对象自身作为对照者检验其“前后”的变化是否显著。其零假设是两配对样本来自的两总体的分布无显著差异。此外，经常应用的还有 x^2 test（卡方检验），它在定性资料分析中可用于两个或多个样本率的比较、两组或多组样本构成比的比较、定性资料的关联分析及频数分布资料的拟合优度检验等。

六、 图片说明

无论是著书立传，还是做科学研究，有时会采用大量的图像或是照片，这不仅让读者对其内容有一个大致的了解，还会为其主题增色。因此，需要作者精心挑选数据库中的精美图像或是照片，在形式上是可以制版的高质量图像；在内容上是不可复制的图像，对主题起画龙点睛之功效。切忌把质量不高，或司空见惯，不能反映主题或者不能明确突出主题的图像放入其中。有些错误的图像，比如：张冠李戴、左右标错、上下颠倒，要严格审查，避免误用。更主要的是，去除图像上所有关于受检者信息的内容，如：姓名、ID 号等。有时为了让读者对图像有更直接的了解，必要时需加箭头引导阅读。

接下来，就是对图像进行必要的说明，文字宜简洁，通常采用就事论事，不要加入主观臆断或修饰性的词句。当图像不能解决问题，或是不能完整表达作者意图时，可以采用多幅图像，分 a, b, c……加以说明。采用多幅图像时，可以用第 1 句概括总体含义，然后再进行分述。

第 121 天

学习

1. Imaging plate(IP) artefact.
   成像板（IP）伪影。
2. Imaging plate reader artefact.
   成像板阅读伪影。
3. Image processing artefact.
   影像处理伪影。
4. Laser printer artefact.
   激光打印伪影。
5. Operator error.
   操作者错误。

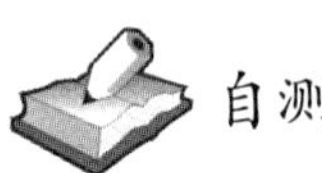
自测

1. 图 1. 影像评价所采用的解剖结构。图 A 和图 B，后前位（A）和侧位（B）X 线照片显

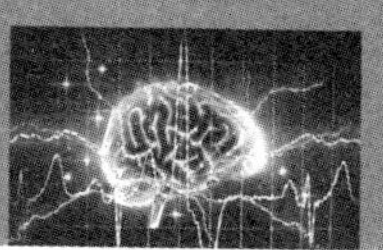

示肺实质（正方形所示）、软组织（箭头所示）及骨骼（长方形所示）。

2. 图 2. 曝光后获得胸部体模 X 线摄影照片，（a）X 形铅条物体证实记忆伪影可出现在多幅影像中。（b、c）在 a 图像曝光后间隔 1min 获取胸部体模影像。这类伪影很少出现在 c 图像中，归究于硒探测器的恢复。

答案

1. Figure 1. Anatomic structures used for image evaluation.A and B.Posteroanterior(A) and lateral(B) radiographs show lung parenchyma(squares),soft tissue(arrows),and bone(rectangle).

2. Figure2. Radiographs of a chest phantom obtained after exposure of(a) a lead X-shaped object demonstrate that the memory artifact can appear in multiple images.(b,c) Chest phantom images were acquired at 1-minute intervals after a.The artifact is less prominent in c owing to recovery of the selenium receptor.

第 122 天

学习

1. Figure 3. Photograph shows flat-panel digital radiography system.
   图 3 照片显示平板数字 X 线摄影系统。
2. Figure 4. Frequency distribution of absorbed doses.
   图 4 吸收剂量的频度分布。
   absorbed doses 吸收剂量

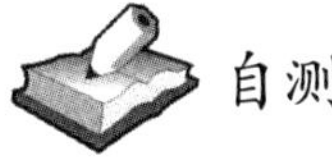

自测

1. 图 5. 轴位骨盆图 a T1 加权脂肪抑制和图 b 双回波 Dixon 磁共振图像显示右侧附件子宫肌瘤（箭头所示）。2 名观察者都判断双回波 Dixon 图像质量更好。

2. 图 6. 容积采集 GRE 图像采用 1.5 mm 层厚，在闭口位时证实关节盘前移，而采用 Burnett 器件同样的位置则没有显示。

答案

1. Figure 5. Axial(a)T1-weighted fat-suppressed and(b) dual-echo Dixon MR images of pelvis show right adnexal endometrioma(arrow).Both readers judged image quality to be better on dual-echo Dixon image.
   adnexal［ æd'neksəl ］*a.* 附件的

endometrioma [ˌendəu'mi:triˌəusis] *n.* 子宫肌瘤

2. Fig.6. Volume acquired GRE image with 1.5mm thickness in the closed mouth position demonstrates anterior displacement of the disk not evident with the Burnett device in place.

七、 表格的建立与说明

科技论文中大多数的表格是建立在统计学基础之上的，为各类研究给读者一个醒目的对比结果。因此，这里面的数据往往是二次加工的结果。所以，表格要考虑建立在数据的科学、直观显示的基础之上，还得考虑读者的易接受性与表格美观。目前，国际上科研论文的表格往往采用三线式，由标识、标题、项目、内容、备注所组成。所涉及英文单词要统一大小写。因词语表达过长时可采用缩略词，然后在表格下就此进行备注。在数字的选取上，往往采用统一的保留小数点后的多少位数。

第 123 天

学习

TABLE 1 Receiver Operating Characteristic(ROC) Analysis of Digital Versus Conventional Radiography

Criteria	Digital Radiography		Conventional Radiography		Difference	
	Area	95%Confidence Interval[a]	Area	95%Confidence Interval	Area	95%Confidence Interval
Chest wall abnormalities	0.7	0.6 ~ 0.8	0.7	0.7 ~ 0.8	-0.1	-0.1 ~ 0.2
Pulmonary nodules	0.9	0.8 ~ 0.9	0.9	0.8 ~ 0.9	0.1	-0.1 ~ 0.2
Mediastinal masses	0.7	0.7 ~ 0.8	0.7	0.6 ~ 0.8	0.1	-0.1 ~ 0.2

[a] 95% Confidence Interval of the area under the ROC curve.

表 1 数字与传统 X 线摄影相比的 ROC 分析

标准	数字 X 线摄影		传统 X 线摄影		差异	
	面积	95% 可信区间[a]	面积	95% 可信区间	面积	95% 可信区间
胸壁异常	0.7	0.6 ~ 0.8	0.7	0.7 ~ 0.8	-0.1	-0.1 ~ 0.2
肺结节	0.9	0.8 ~ 0.9	0.9	0.8 ~ 0.9	0.1	-0.1 ~ 0.2

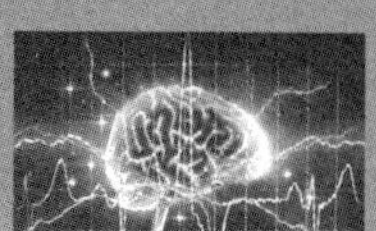

续表

标准	数字 X 线摄影		传统 X 线摄影		差异	
	面积	95% 可信区间[a]	面积	95% 可信区间	面积	95% 可信区间
纵隔肿块	0.7	0.7 ~ 0.8	0.7	0.6 ~ 0.8	0.1	−0.1 ~ 0.2

[a] 95% 可信区间的 ROC 曲线下面积。

confidence interval 可信区间

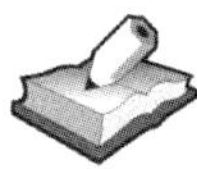

自测

表 2　对患者检查采用相同曝光剂量进行胸部前后位体模的剂量测试

参数	成像系统	
	数字	屏 - 片
感光度	400	200
峰电压	125	125
毫安	160	395
毫安秒	2.16	5.1
表面剂量	132	259
剂量下降（%）	50.1	

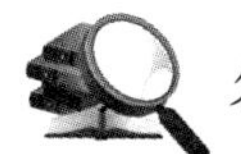

答案

TABLE 2　Dose Measurements with Anthropomorphic Chest Phantom Using Same Exposure as for Patient Examinations

Parameter	Imaging System	
	Digital	Film-Screen
Speed	400	200
Peak kilovoltage	125	125
Milliamperage	160	395
Milliampere-seconds	2.16	5.1
Surface dose(mGy)	132	259
Dose reduction（%）	50.1	

peak kilovoltage 峰电压

第 124 天

TABLE 3　Quality of Radiographs Obtained with Digital and Conventional Radiography Systems

Image Quality of	Imaging System		Δ	P
	Digital	Film-Screen		
Posteroanterior radiographs	4.1(0.7)	3.7(0.7)	0.4	0.1
Lateral radiographs	3.9(0.7)	3.5(0.7)	0.4	0.1

Note:Data are mean ± SD of scores for image quality evaluated using a 5-point scale(1=unsatisfactory, 2=poor, 3=fair, 4=good, 5=excellent). Δ =difference of mean scores.

表 3　采用数字和传统 X 线摄影系统所获得的照片质量

影像质量	成像系统		Δ	P
	数字	屏 - 片		
后前位 X 线照片	4.1(0.7)	3.7(0.7)	0.4	0.1
侧位 X 线照片	3.9(0.7)	3.5(0.7)	0.4	0.1

注：分数均值 ± SD 的影像质量评价采用 5 分制（1= 不满意，2= 不好，3= 一般，4= 好，5= 优秀）。Δ = 均值分数的差异。

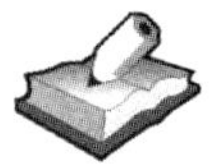

表 4　数字图像与传统胶片图像对异常的一致性

观察者	K 统计加权	95% 可信区间
1	0.8	0.6，0.9
2	0.7	0.5，0.9
3	0.7	0.5，0.9
4	0.5	0.3，0.8

TABLE 4　Level of Agreement Between Digital and Conventional Film Images for Presence of Abnormality

Observer	Weighted Kappa Statistic	95% Confidence Interval
1	0.8	0.6，0.9
2	0.7	0.5，0.9

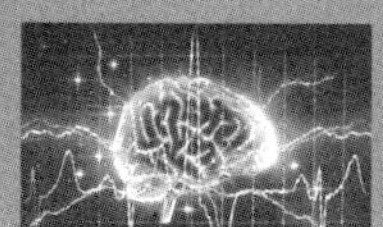

续表

Observer	Weighted Kappa Statistic	95% Confidence Interval
3	0.7	0.5，0.9
4	0.5	0.3，0.8

第 125 天

学习

Table 5　The total percentage of studies that were deemed to be diagnostic by each observer for each group

% of studies that were diagnostic	All traditional IVUs(%)	traditional IVUs with conventional tomography(%)	Digital tomosynthesis(%)
Observer 1	48	54	99
Observer 2	45	62	92
Average of 2 observers	46.5	58	95.5

Note:IVU, intravenous urogram.

表 5　各组每位观察者诊断研究的百分数

诊断研究的百分数	传统 IVU（%）	传统 IVU 与传统体层摄影（%）	数字融合体层摄影
观察者 1	48	54	99
观察者 2	45	62	92
2 位观察者的平均	46.5	58	95.5

注：IVU 为静脉肾盂造影。

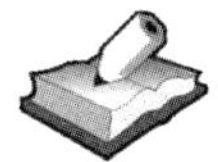
自测

表 6　计算机 X 线摄影 (CR) 与数字 X 线摄影 (DR) 对于单幅图像检查的时间

工作流程 CR	平均时间 (s)	标准差 (s)	DR 平均时间 (s)	标准差 (s)	平均时间差异 (s)
检查准备	19.8	4.8	19.4	6.0	0.4
病人定位	32.2	11.8	30.8	13.0	1.4
曝光	2.4	1.3	4.3	1.8	-1.9
后处理	51.0	9.6	24.4	5.7	26.6
整个检查	105.4	17.7	78.9	15.8	26.4

答案

TABLE 6 Computed Radiography(CR) and Digital Radiography(DR) Times for Single-View Radiographic Examinations

Workflow Segment	Mean CR Time(s)	SD(s)	Mean DR Time(s)	SD(s)	Mean Time Difference(s)
Examination preparation	19.8	4.8	19.4	6.0	0.4
Patient positioning	32.2	11.8	30.8	13.0	1.4
Exposure	2.4	1.3	4.3	1.8	-1.9
Postacquisition processing	51.0	9.6	24.4	5.7	26.6
Entire examination	105.4	17.7	78.9	15.8	26.4

第 126 天

学习

Table 7 CT Effective Dose Estimates Based on Anatomic Coverage Region

Covered Anatomy	Assigned Effective Dose per CT Examination(mSv)
Head,face	2
Cervical spine,neck	2
Chest,pulmonary embolus,thoracic spine	8
Abdomen alone(no pelvis)	7.5
Pelvis alone(no abdomen)	7.5
Abdomen and pelvis,lumbar spine	15
Extremity	0

表 7 基于解剖覆盖区域 CT 有效剂量评估

覆盖的解剖部位	每次 CT 检查所得有效剂量 (mSv)
头颅、面部	2
颈髓，颈部	2
胸部，肺动脉栓塞，胸髓	8
腹部（不含骨盆）	7.5
骨盆（不含腹部）	7.5
腹部与骨盆，腰髓	15
四肢	0

cervical spine 颈髓　　thoracic spine 胸髓

lumbar spine 腰髓　　pulmonary embolus 肺动脉栓塞

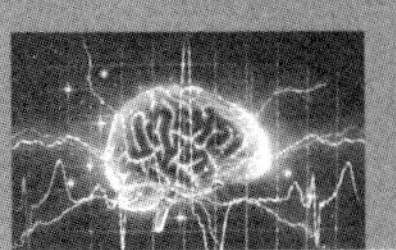

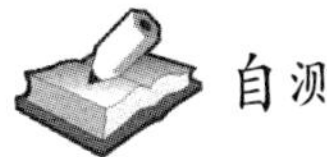
自测

1.

表 8　64 层 CT 协议参数

参数	头颅 CT	3D CT 血管成像
千伏 (kV)	120	120
管电流 (mA)	250	300
旋转时间 (s)	1.0	0.5
螺距	间断扫描	0.61
轴位层厚 (mm)	4 and 8	0.5
重建间隔 (mm)	4 and 8	0.4

2.

表 9　所有观察者与所有结构在传统胶片与数字图像之间的差异

结构	均值	*P* 值	显著差异
肺	−0.68	<0.000 1	Yes[a]
线型结构	−0.43	<0.000 1	Yes[a]
钙化	−0.04	<0.45	No
囊肿	−0.65	<0.005	Yes[a]
皮肤表面	+0.83	<0.000 1	Yes[b]

[a] 传统胶片比数字图像好。
[b] 数字图像比传统胶片好。

答案

1.

Table 8　64–slice CT protocol parameters

Parameter	头颅 CT	3D CT 血管成像
Tube voltage(kV)	120	120
Tube current(mA)	250	300
Rotation time(s)	1.0	0.5
Pitch	Incremental	0.61
Axial section thickness(mm)	4 and 8	0.5
Reconstruction interval(mm)	4 and 8	0.4

2. Table 9 Difference(significant deviation from 0)between the conventional films and digital images for all observers and all structures

Structure	Mean	*P*-value	Significance of difference
Parenchyma	−0.68	<0.000 1	Yes[a]
Linear structures	−0.43	<0.000 1	Yes[a]
Calcification	−0.04	<0.45	No
Cyst	−0.65	<0.005	Yes[a]
Skin surface	+0.83	<0.000 1	Yes[b]

[a] The conventional film is better than the digital image.

[b] The digital image is better than the conventional film.

八、 增设小标题

有时为了能让读者清晰地了解作者写作意图与内涵，或是为了做到层层递进，长篇大论中往往需要增设若干个小标题，对下面段落起提纲挈领的作用。而这类小标题往往只是标题式的，以核心词汇构成，甚至称得上是“关键词”，而不是句子，因此无需标点符号。

第 127 天

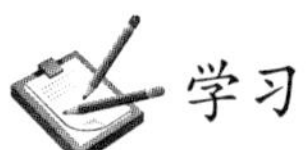
学习

Digital Radiography

数字 X 线摄影

Conventional Radiography

传统 X 线摄影

Image Evaluation

影像评价

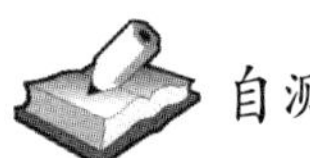
自测

与参考标准相比数字和传统 X 线摄影的判断

与传统 X 线摄影相比数字 X 线摄影的 ROC 分析

ROC 分析中观察者间的变化

答案

Digtal Conventional Radiography Ratings versus the Reference Standard

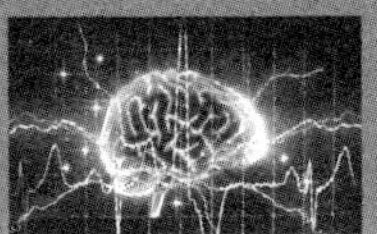

ROC Analysis of Digital versus Conventional Radiography

Interobserver Variability for the ROC Analysis

第 128 天

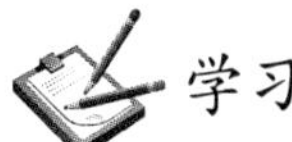

学习

Patients

MRI

Image Analysis

Statistical Analysis

患者

磁共振成像

影像分析

统计分析

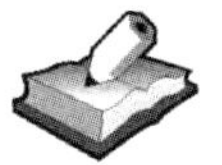

自测

患者

成像系统

剂量测试

影像评价

答案

Patients

Imaging Systems

Dose Measurements

Image Evaluation

第 129 天

学习

1. Patients

   Dual-Source CT Scanning

   Tube Voltage and Estimation of Effective Dose

Assessment of Image Quality
Statistical Analysis
患者
双源 CT 扫描
管电压和有效剂量评估
图像质量评价
统计学分析

2. Sensitivity
Specificity
ROC analysis
Radiology
灵敏度
特异性
受试者作业特征曲线（ROC）分析
放射学

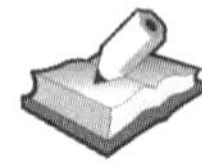 自测

引言
灵敏度与特异性：需要 ROC 分析
ROC 曲线：基本原理
ROC 分析的实际应用
ROC 分析的应用：比较测试与观察者
ROC 分析的应用：最佳阈值

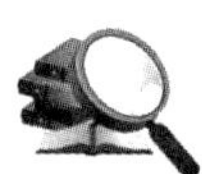 答案

Introduction
Sensitivity and specificity:need for ROC analysis
The ROC curve:basic principles
Practical aspects of ROC analysis
Applications of ROC analysis:comparing tests or observers
Applications of ROC analysis:optimizing the threshold value

九、 伦理道德

以上所有研究如果是利用人来进行，则必须要向受试者讲明作者所需研究的利弊关系，

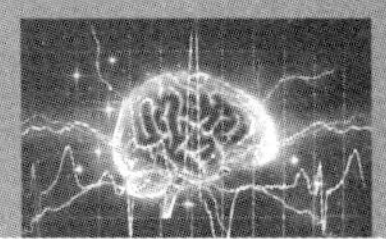

特别是对受试者的危害不能隐瞒；即使是利用现成的资料，对受试者没有利害冲突，也要征得受试者同意才可把他（她）的相关资料用于科学研究；受试者知情并同意后签字，作者还须征得相关部门如伦理委员会的同意方可实施其科学研究。

第 130 天

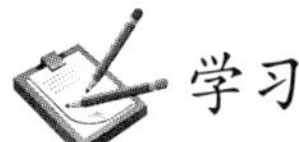

学习

Institutional review board approval was obtained before beginning the evaluation.

在开始评价之前获得研究所伦理委员会的同意。

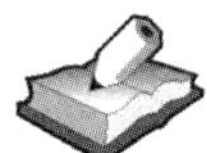

自测

此次实验经伦理委员会批准，并征得患者书面同意。

答案

Institutional review board approval and written informed patient consent were obtained.

第 131 天

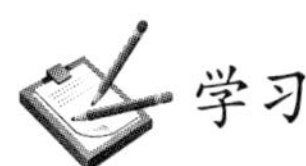

学习

Written consent was obtained from each patient and the study was approved by the institutional review board before digital radiographs were obtained.

本研究是在得到每一个患者的签字同意及学院伦理委员会批准后摄取患者的数字 X 线影像的。

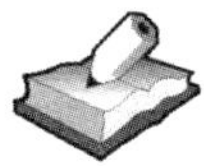

自测

根据 Zurich 大学的伦理委员会制定的规定，在得到参与患者知情并同意后才能展开这项研究。

答案

All patients must give informed consent for this study in accordance with regulations set forth by the institutional review board of the University of Zurich.

第 132 天

 学习

This protocol was approved by the Asian Medical Center institutional review board. Informed consent was obtained from all subjects after they were informed about the use of Xe gas and the DE technique of dual-source CT.

这项方案被亚洲医学中心机构伦理委员会批准。Xe 和双源 CT 的双能量技术的使用是经过研究对象同意的。

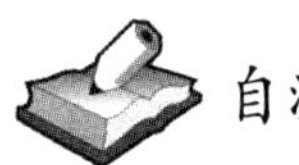 自测

我们的研究方案是经过当地伦理委员会认可，同时我们已经将本次放射剂量信息上交给该委员会。所有的患者在同意参加本次研究前都被告知放射剂量信息。

 答案

Our study protocol was approved by the local Ethics Committee, with radiation dose information having been submitted to that Committee. All patients provided informed consent for participation in the study after having been informed of radiation dose information.

ethics ['eθiks] *n.* 伦理　　committee [kə'miti] *n.* 委员会

submit [səb'mit] *v.* 提交；be submitted to 送请、已提交；I submit that... 我认为……

第 133 天

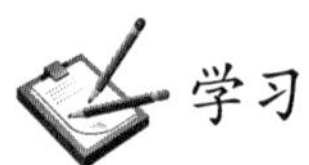 学习

At the time our study was conducted, our ethics committee did not require its approval or patient-informed consent, because patient's reports had been based on hard-copy interpretation, and soft-copy interpretation was not yet routinely used in our department for projection radiography. The study setup was in agreement with the *Helsinki Declaration*, according to which all patient-related information (such as name and identification number) was obscured during interpretation.

我们的研究无须伦理委员会批准或患者告知书的认可，因为患者的报告基于硬拷贝判读，在我们科软拷贝判读还没有常规使用。根据《赫尔辛基宣言》本研究在判读时隐去患者相关信息（如姓名或身份证号）。

Helsinki ['helsiŋki] *n.* 赫尔辛基（芬兰首都）

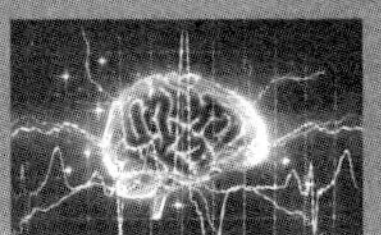

Helsinki Declaration《赫尔辛基宣言》

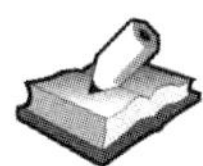 自测

根据政府公布的法律，医院伦理委员会基于医院保护患者隐私的政策公布了一份回顾性观察图像数据的许可证。该政策包括患者享有拒绝自己的图像数据用于科学研究的权利。

 答案

In accordance with applicable state law, the hospital's institutional review board has issued a general permit for retrospective review of image data based on the hospital's policy protecting the patient's privacy, which includes the patiens' right to reject the use of their image data for scientific purposes.

十、 不足之处

最后，可适当地阐述作者在研究过程中不可避免的一些问题，或是因客观条件所致的一些不足之处。

第 134 天

 学习

Dose measurements for the patient examinations were not performed.
对患者检查没有进行剂量测试。

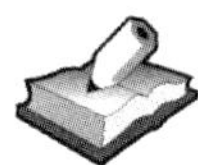 自测

患者确切的入射剂量没有测量。

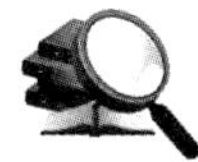 答案

However, the exact entrance exposure for patients was not measured.

第 135 天

Because the digital images could be distinguished visually from the film-screen images, a blinded study could not be performed.

因为数字影像在目视下可与屏 - 片成像区别，所以双盲研究不能进行。

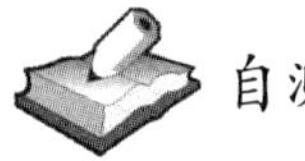

尽管数字和传统影像不被标示，但是由于传统和激光 X 线照片的特性它们还是容易被区分出来。

Digital and conventional images were not identified, but could be easily recognized because of the specific properties of conventional and laser radiographs.

第 136 天

Because neither technique can be regarded as the gold standard in this case, our analysis is not an analysis of accuracy but to provide some indication of the level of consistency between digital and film images with respect to diagnosis.

因为没有一种技术被当作金标准，所以我们的分析不是一种精确性分析，而是为了证实数字与屏 - 片成像之间关于诊断问题的一致性水平。

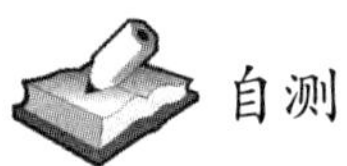

硒数字 X 线成像采用 2 560 × 3 072 矩阵及 8 bit 灰阶的激光相机。用可取的算法在 35 cm × 43 cm 的胶片上激光打印，在目测情况下，由于片基的不同色调，激光打印硒数字 X 线成像的图像可与屏 - 片成像区别。传统胶片大小为 23.5 cm × 29.5 cm。

Selenium-based digital radiographic images were laser-printed with the preferred algorithms on 35 cm × 43 cm film using a laser camera with a 2 560 × 3 072 matrix and an 8 bit gray scale.

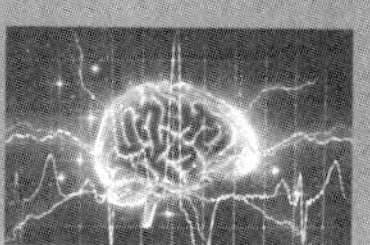

The laser-printed selenium-based digital radiographic images could be visually distinguished from film-screen images by the different color of the film base. The conventional films measured 23.5 cm × 29.5 cm.

十一、结果与讨论

结果是根据前面所述的科研方法得出客观的数据，尤其要有统计学数据，要通过统计量来表现结果，尽量做到确切、具体、客观、定量的描述。不可笼统地用 $P < 0.05$ 或 $P > 0.01$ 表示，更不能抽象地主观评价和阐述。要通过统计学表达作者在资料选择上是否存在差异，观察者之间是否存在差异；要通过统计学体现受试者总体上是否存在差异，组间是否存在差异。在结果中一定要尊重事实，对于个性问题可以单列，如实反映研究产生的差异，这可以留在讨论中阐述其产生共性与个性的原因。总之，结果是对研究所得的原始数据进行科学的归纳和统计学处理的最终体现。

第 137 天

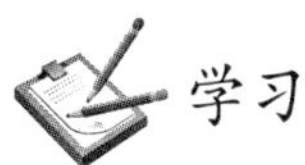

学习

The visibility of all but one anatomic structure on the images obtained with the digital system was rated significantly superior to the images obtained with the reference film-screen system. One exception was the basal peripheral lung vessels in the posteroanterior view. An insignificant advantage was noted for the digital system for these structures.

在用数字系统所获得的影像上，除 1 个解剖结构外，所有解剖结构的显示能力显著优于屏 - 片系统所获得的影像。这个例外是在后前位中的外周肺血管。对于这些结构数字系统无显著优势。

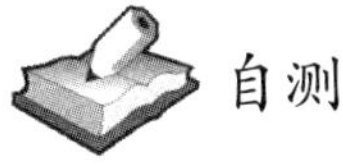

自测

在评价影像质量中，这 3 种成像显示方法间无明显的统计学差异。但与硬拷贝胶片或 LCD 显示器上的软拷贝影像相比，经验少的放射学家更喜欢高分辨率软拷贝图像。

答案

In evaluating image quality, no statistically significant difference was seen among the three imaging display methods. However, less experienced radiologists seemed to prefer the soft-copy images on the high-resolution video monitor compared with hard-copy film or soft-copy images viewed on the LCD monitor.

第 138 天

学习

Average ovarian dose was low (0.21—0.37 mGy) among all the scan protocols. Average ovarian radiation dose from the standard helical plus axial HRCT scans was slightly greater by 0.12 mGy (25%) than dose from the combination helical scan alone ($P < 0.01$).

在所有扫描方案中，卵巢的平均剂量低（0.21 ~ 0.37 mGy）。来自于标准螺旋加轴位 HRCT 扫描的卵巢的平均放射剂量要比单一的组合螺旋扫描略高 0.12 mGy（25%）（$P < 0.01$）。

ovarian [əu'vɛəriən] *a.* 卵巢的

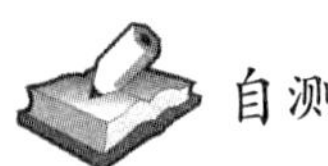

自测

根据整体印象，采用低探测器剂量（1.8 μGy）所获得的影像比用标准剂量（2.5 μGy）所获得的影像略好。但是，此种差异是非常小的，且无统计学意义。整个较小的标准差证实观察者间几乎没有偏差。放射学家的结论和其他观察者所得到的结果没有明显差异。

答案

According to the overall impression, the images obtained with the reduced detector dose (1.8 μGy) were rated slightly better than those obtained with standard dose (2.5 μGy). However, this difference is very small and not statistically significant. The overall small standard deviations indicate little interobserver variability. None of the radiologists presented results that were consistently different from those of other observers.

第 139 天

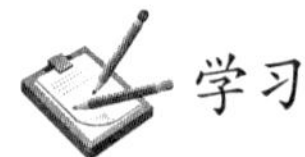

学习

Image quality was significantly better in patients with low heart rates than in patients with high heart rates (relative timing: $r = 0.98$, $P < 0.01$; absolute timing: $r = 0.93$, $P < 0.01$), showing no significant differences between relative and absolute timing.

低心率患者的图像质量明显好于高心率者（相对时间：$r = 0.98$, $P < 0 .01$；绝对时间：$r = 0.93$, $P < 0.01$），相对时间和绝对时间无显著差异。

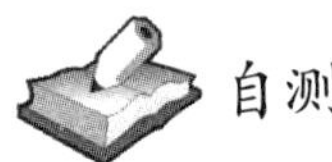

自测

数据的统计学分析（t 检验）也显示光学密度为 0.90 的胶片（P=0.34）与遮蔽胶片没有

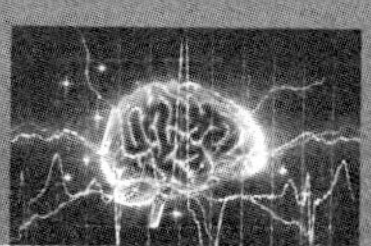

显著差异。但对于 1.83 和 2.27 的胶片密度（$P < 0.01$）遮蔽的作用是显著的。

 答案

Statistical analysis (*t* test) of the data also shows that film masking makes no significant difference for film with an optical density of 0.90 (P=0.34). However, the effect of masking is significant for film densities of 1.83 and 2.27($P < 0.01$).

第 140 天

 学习

For soft-tissue assessment, four of five observers found digital and film imaging to be equivalent with respect to image quality. The fifth observer, for whom equivalence could not be established, found digital image quality superior to that of film (mean difference, 0.92 rating units). For one of the observers who found digital and film image quality to be equivalent, the average image quality for digital imaging was significantly greater than that for film-screen (mean difference, 0.64 rating units).

对于软组织的评价，5 位观察者中有 4 位发现关于影像质量数字与屏 - 片成像是等同的。第 5 位观察者不这样认为，他发现数字影像质量优于屏 - 片成像（平均差为 0.92 评价单位）。对于发现数字与屏 - 片成像质量等同的 4 位中的 1 位来说，数字成像的平均影像质量比屏 - 片成像明显高（平均差为 0.64 评价单位）。

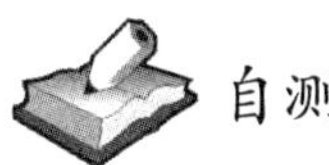 自测

对于骨骼结构，这两种 X 线摄影系统之间观察的最大差异表现在后前位上胸椎脊突的显示能力。对于这些结构数字影像的平均得分为 3.38，而屏 - 片 X 线摄影系统的影像为 3.09（△ =0.29）。对于大多数解剖结构，Spearman 秩相关显示观察者间有显著的一致性。

 答案

For the bony structures, the biggest differences between the two radiography systems were observed for the visibility of the pedicles of the upper thoracic spine on the posteroanterior view. For these structures, the mean score of the digital images was 3.38, compared with 3.09 for the images of the film-screen radiography system (△ = 0.29). For most anatomic structures, a significant interobserver agreement was shown by the Spearman's rank correlation.

pedicle ['pedikl] *n.* 蒂　　　bony ['bəuni] *a.* 骨的

第 141 天

学习

Central chest and breast radiation dose was lower from the standard helical chest plus axial HRCT when compared with the combination helical protocol alone. Radiation exposure was lower by an average of 11.69 mGy (33%) in the central chests ($P = 0.001$) and an average of 7.46 mGy (25%) in the breasts($P < 0.05$). Total TLD measured radiation dose was higher from the combination helical protocol compared with the standard helical plus axial HRCT protocols by 32% ($P < 0.001$).

与组合螺旋方案比较，胸部中间位置和乳腺吸收剂量要低于标准螺旋胸部加轴位 HRCT 扫描。在胸部中间位置（$P=0.001$）辐射曝光剂量平均低于 11.69 mGy（33%），乳腺位置（$P < 0.05$）平均低于 7.46 mGy（25%）。与标准螺旋加轴位 HRCT 扫描相比，组合螺旋方案的 TLD 的总测量放射剂量要高 32%（$P < 0.001$）。

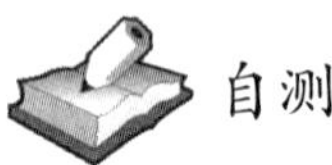

自测

我们从两个由传统 X 线片构成的远程放射学研究，以及一个包括传统 X 线照片与 CT 扫描的研究中综合考虑差异率以判定我们的差异率是否具有显著性。这三项研究的综合差异率是 3%。我们的数据资料与采用二项式检验的这三项研究数据比较表明无明显的统计学差异（$P < 0.25$）。

答案

We combined the discrepancy rates from two teleradiology studies comprised of conventional radiographs and one study that included conventional radiographs and CT scans to determine whether our discrepancy rate was significantly different. The combined discrepancy rate of these three studies was 3%. The comparison of our data with those from these three studies using a binomial test revealed no statistically significant difference ($P < 0.25$).

discrepancy [dis'krepəsi] *n.* 不同、差异　　　binomial [bai'nəumiəl] *n.* 二项式

第 142 天

学习

For cortical bone, three of five observers found digital and film imaging to be equivalent with respect to image quality. Both of the observers for whom equivalence could not be established

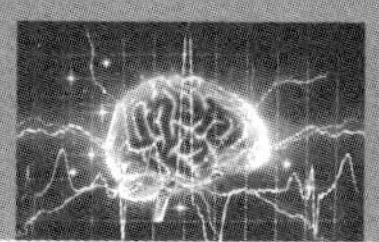

found digital image quality superior to that of film (mean difference, 0.84 rating units in both cases). For one of the observers who found digital and film image quality to be equivalent, the average image quality for digital imaging was significantly greater than for film-screen (mean difference, 0.56 rating units).

关于骨皮质，5 位观察者中的 3 位发现数字与屏 - 片成像的影像质量相当。观察者中的 2 位并不这么认为，他们发现数字成像质量优于屏 - 片成像（平均差为 0.84 评价单位）。发现数字与屏 - 片成像质量相当的 3 位观察者中的 1 位认为，数字成像平均影像质量比屏 - 片成像明显高（平均差为 0.56 评价单位）。

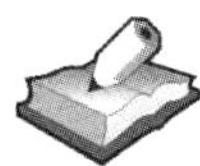自测

关于骨小梁，5 位观察者中的 3 位发现数字与屏 - 片成像影像质量相当。5 位观察者中的 2 位不认为相当，他们发现数字影像质量优于屏 - 片成像（一个平均差为 0.68，另一个为 0.80）。发现数字与屏 - 片成像质量相当的 5 位观察者中的 2 位，认为数字影像的平均影像质量比屏 - 片成像明显高（平均差为 0.72 及 0.48）。

答案

For trabecular bone, three of five observers found digital and film imaging to be equivalent with respect to image quality. Both of the observers for whom equivalence could not be established found digital image quality superior to that of film (mean difference, 0.68 rating units in one case and 0.80 in the other). For two of the observers who found digital and film image quality to be equivalent, the average image quality for digital imaging was significantly greater than that for film-screen (mean difference, 0.72 and 0.48 rating units).

trabecula [trə'bekjulə] *n.* 小梁；复数 trabeculae [trə'bekjuli:]

第 143 天

学习

Four of five observers found digital and film imaging to be equivalent with respect to overall image quality. The observer for whom equivalence could not be established found digital image quality superior to that of film (mean difference, 0.72 rating units). For two of the observers who found digital and film image quality to be equivalent, the average image quality for digital imaging was significantly greater than that for film-screen (mean differences, 0.64 and 0.52 rating units).

5 位观察者中的 4 位发现数字及屏 - 片成像的整体影像质量相当。认为不相当的观察

者发现数字成像质量优于屏 - 片成像(平均差为 0.72)。发现数字及屏 - 片成像质量相当的观察者中的 2 位认为数字成像的平均影像质量比屏 - 片成像明显高(平均差异为 0.64，0.52)。

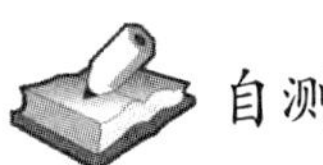

自测

关于通常的 mAs 值，后前位图像降低了 24%(0.85 mAs 与 31.12 mAs)，侧位图像下降了 35%(3.054 mAs 与 4.697 mAs)，导致整体下降了 33%(3.904 mAs 与 35.817 mAs)。侧位图像的 mAs 值比后前位摄影的 mAs 值要高得多。这是由于在侧位胸部 X 线照片中放射线既要穿过两边的肺，又要穿过纵隔，而正位 X 线照片仅穿过一个肺或仅穿过纵隔即可。

答案

As for the average milliampere-second values, a reduction of 24% (0.85 vs 1.12 mAs) for posteroanterior and 35% (3.054 vs 4.697 mAs) for lateral views was achieved, resulting in a total reduction of 33% (3.904 vs 5.817 mAs). The milliampere-second values of the lateral views were much higher than those of the posteroanterior projections. This finding reflects the fact that radiation has to penetrate both lungs and the mediastinum in the lateral chest radiographs as opposed to having to penetrate only one lung or the mediastinum in the frontal radiographs.

milliampere-second 毫安秒　　penetrate ['penitreit] *v.* 透入、贯穿

frontal ['frʌntl] *n.* 正面、前面

第 144 天

学习

For the lung parenchyma structures, the biggest difference noted between the two systems was the visibility of the small lung vessels in the retrocardiac space on the lateral view. The mean score for the digital images of this structure was 3.73, compared with 3.09 of the conventional film-screen images (△ = 0.64). For the soft-tissue structures, the biggest differences between the two radiography systems were observed for the delineation of the diaphragm in the posteroanterior view. The mean score for the digital images of this structure was 4.03, compared with 3.54 for the film-screen system (△ = 0.49).

对于肺实质结构，这两种系统间的最大差异表现在侧位心后间隙的小的肺血管的显示能力。此结构的数字影像平均得分为 3.73，而传统屏 - 片影像为 3.09(△ =0.64)。对于软组织结构，为后前位片上横膈的描述观察两种 X 线摄影系统间的最大差异。此结构的数字影像平均得分为 4.03，屏 - 片系统为 3.54(△ =0.49)。

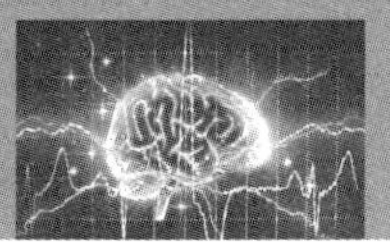

parenchyma [pə'reŋkimə] *n.* 实质　　　retrocardiac [retrəu'kɑ:diæk] *a.* 心后的

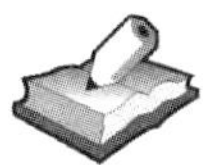

自测

从 137 个头颅的连续 CT 扫描中,在 66 例(48%)中至少有 1 位观察者发现异常,指出有疾病或损伤;在 71 例(52%)中,没有观察者发现疾病或损伤征象。放射学家对其中 118 例 (86%) 的判读是一致的。14 例(10%)的判读结果不同,但我们认为差异是微小的。把完全一致的结果及微小差异的结果结合起来看,我们的方法获得 96% 的一致性。5 例(4%)产生较大差异。

答案

From the 137 consecutive CT scans of the head, at least one observer detected findings indicating disease or injury in 66 cases (48%), and neither observer found indications of disease or injury in 71 cases (52%). On 118 studies (86%) the radiologists' interpretations were the same. In 14 cases (10%) interpretations differed but differences were thought to be minor. Combining complete agreements with minor discrepancies, our method achieved a 96% concordance. Five cases (4%) yielded major discrepancies.

concordance [kən'kɔ:dəns] *n.* 一致、协调

第 145 天

学习

For detecting urinary calculi, the paired *t* test did not show a statistically significant difference between the soft-copy display and the hard-copy format. In the soft-copy display, no statistically significant difference was seen in the various display systems—the high resolution versus the LCD monitor. However, each of the radiologists performed well when viewing images from the soft-copy display compared with viewing them from the hard-copy films. Although not statistically significant, the overall performance of the radiologists was also better with the soft-copy display. This improved performance was more conspicuous in the less experienced than in the more experienced radiologists.

对于诊断泌尿系结石,软拷贝显示与硬拷贝格式间配对 *t* 检验未显示明显的统计学差异。在软拷贝显示中,不同的显示系统,即高分辨率(high resolution, HR)显示器与液晶显示器(liquid crystal display, LCD)之间无明显的统计学差异。但放射学家从软拷贝观看显示的影像效果好于从硬拷贝胶片观看影像。尽管无显著性差异,放射学家利用软拷贝显示总体性能更好。经验少的放射学家比经验丰富的放射学家改善更显著。

conspicuous [kən'spikjuəs] *a.* 显著的、明显的

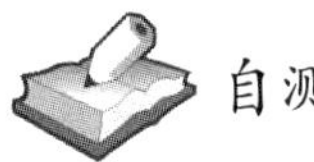

自测

总共对 2 800 个数据集进行了重建。研究人员的评分一致率在基于相对时间重建的图像中达 0.71 (95% *CI*: 0.65, 0.77),基于绝对时间重建图像中达 0.94 (95% *CI*: 0.92, 0.95)。由于这些结论被视为好和优秀,其后所有的计算结果与数据均采用了双方的评价数据。基于绝对时间的图像重建显著 ($P < 0.001$) (2.4) 优于基于相对时间的图像重建 (2.6); 图像质量平均差异为 0.20 (95% *CI*: 0.15, 0.23)。

答案

In total, 2 800 data sets were reconstructed. The strength of agreement between the observers in the grading of reconstruction intervals amounted to 0.71 (95% *CI*: 0.65, 0.77) for image reconstruction based on relative timing and 0.94 (95% *CI*: 0.92, 0.95) for image reconstruction based on absolute timing. Since these agreements were regarded as excellent and very good, respectively, all subsequent calculations were performed with the pooled data of both investigators. Image reconstruction based on absolute timing was significantly ($P < 0.001$) better (ie, 2.4) than image reconstruction based on relative timing (ie, 2.6); image quality differed by 0.20 grading point (95% *CI*: 0.15, 0.23), on average.

第 146 天

学习

The quality of the images obtained with the digital flat-panel detector system was rated significantly superior to the quality of those obtained with the conventional film-screen radiography system. The mean scores for the image quality of the digital images were 4.11 and 3.93 (posteroanterior and lateral views, respectively) compared with 3.74 and 3.51 for the film-screen images. The difference (Δ)of the mean scores between the two systems for the image quality was 0.37 and 0.42 (posteroanterior and lateral views, respectively). For the image quality, a significant interobserver agreement was shown by the Spearman's rank correlation ($P \leqslant 0.02$).

我们用数字平板探测器系统所获得的影像质量等级明显优于用传统屏 - 片 X 线摄影系统所获得的影像质量。数字图像的影像质量平均得分是 4.11 和 3.93 (分别为后前位和侧位),而屏 - 片图像质量则分别为 3.74 和 3.51。两种系统间影像质量均差为 0.37 和 0.42 (分别为后前位和侧位)。通过 Spearman 秩相关显示观察者间对于影像质量显著的一致 ($P \leqslant 0.02$)。

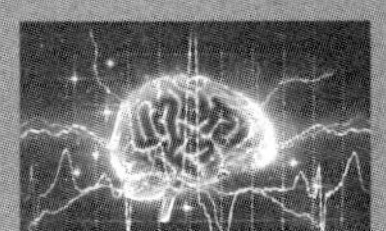

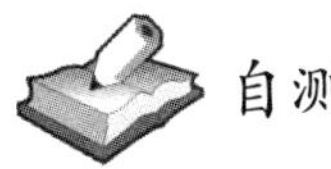

自测

在我们的病例中,基于部分的分析显示的总体准确率是 91.9%(1 229 中的 1 129)。总的敏感度是 91.1%(259 中的 236),特异性为 92.0%(970 中的 893),阳性预测值是 75.4%(313 中的 236),阴性预测值是 97.5%(916 中的 893)。而对每个患者而言,准确率是 95.0%(100 中的 95),敏感度是 100%(73 中的 73),特异性是 81.5%(27 中的 22),阳性预测值是 93.6%(78 中的 73),阴性预测值是 100%(22 中的 22)。

答案

In our collective, overall accuracy on the basis of a per-segment analysis was 91.9% (1 129 of 1 229). Overall sensitivity was 91.1% (236 of 259), specificity was 92.0% (893 of 970), positive predictive value was 75.4% (236 of 313), and negative predictive value was 97.5% (893 of 916). On the basis of a per-patient analysis, accuracy was 95.0% (95 of 100), sensitivity was 100% (73 of 73), specificity was 81.5% (22 of 27), positive predictive value was 93.6% (73 of 78), and negative predictive value was 100% (22 of 22).

positive predictive value 阳性预测值　　negative predictive value 阴性预测值

第 147 天

学习

Statistical analysis (*t* test) shows a significant improvement ($P < 0.01$) in object detection using a masked, brighter (8 000 nit) viewbox compared with an unmasked regular viewbox (＜3 000 nit) for film densities of 1.83 and 2.27. But the improvement is not significant (P=0.14) for a film density of 0.90 (not shown in the graph). As the optical density of the mammography film increases, the improvement becomes more significant. Objects 50% smaller can be visualized on a masked brighter viewbox as compared with an unmasked regular viewbox (at densities of approximately 2.27). The difference in minimum detectable object size can be attributed both to the extraneous light for the unmasked viewbox and to the luminance level difference between two viewboxes.

统计学分析(*t* 检验)显示用遮蔽、明亮(8 000 nit)观片灯比常规、未遮蔽观片灯(＜3 000 nit)对于胶片密度为 1.83 和 2.27 的病灶检出率有显著提高($P < 0.01$)。但对密度为 0.90 的胶片(图中未显示)提高不显著(P=0.14)。当乳腺 X 线摄影胶片光学密度增加时,这种提高变得尤为显著。遮蔽的、比较明亮的观片灯比传统、未遮蔽的观片灯(大约 2.27 的密度)能显示小一半的物体。未遮蔽观片灯的额外光线和 2 个观片灯之间的亮

度差异决定了可发现物体的最小尺寸。

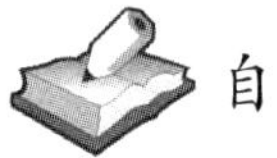

与心率≤ 70/min 的患者相比，心率＞ 70/min 的患者的平均图像质量和移动致使图像质量下降的总数并没有明显的区别（分别为 P=0.13 和 0.37）。在给定 100 份样本大小和各部分图像质量的观测标准差时，这种分析有 94% 的能力诊断平均图像质量差异只有 0.50 之间的差别。根据所有冠状动脉部分的心率对平均图像质量影响的线性回归分析，以及线性回归方程的使用，在心率高达 95.2/min 时仍可获得好的或者优秀的图像质量。

Mean image quality and the total number of motion-degraded segments were not significantly different in patients with heart rates more than 70 beats per minute compared with patients with heart rates 70 or fewer beats per minute (P = 0.13 and 0.37, respectively). Given the sample size of 100 patients and the observed standard deviations in our subgroups for image quality, this analysis had 94% power to detect a difference between the means of image quality of 0.50. According to linear regression analysis of mean image quality for all coronary segments against heart rate and the use of a linear regression equation, good or excellent image quality can be achieved for heart rates up to 95.2 beats per minute.

第 148 天

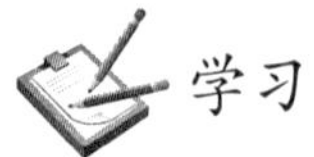

Table 2 shows the differences of the areas under the ROC curves for all the observers. These differences of the area under the ROC curve of the digital radiography minus the corresponding area of the conventional radiography range from 0.064 (mediastinal abnormalities) to −0.023 (calcifications). Regarding these differences for each observer, these quantities differ by less than 0.1 from the quantity which is calculated for all observers. Overall, no large differences among the ratings of the four observers were found. However, the observed area under the ROC curve for mediastinal abnormalities for the digital method was greater than the corresponding area for the conventional method for observer 1 (difference = 0.079), observer 2 (difference = 0.103), and observer 3 (difference = 0.091), whereas the opposite was true for observer 4 (difference = −0.025).

表 2 显示所有观察者 ROC 曲线下区域的差异。数字 X 线摄影 ROC 曲线下的区域减去传统 X 线摄影的相应区域的这些差异范围从 0.064（纵隔异常）到 −0.023（钙化）。对每个

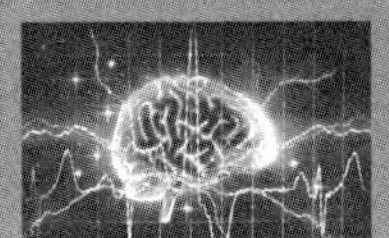

观察者来说，这些差别与所有观察者的总量的差别不到 0.1。总之，4 位观察者的发现率没有大的差异。而对于数字方法，其纵隔异常 ROC 曲线下的观察区域比传统方法的相关区域差异要大些，观察者 1 差异为 0.079，观察者 2 差异为 0.103，观察者 3 差异为 0.091，而观察者 4 则相反，为 -0.025。

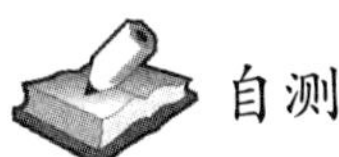

自测

ROC 曲线下的区域依据不同的标准而定，其范围从 0.687（纵隔异常，传统方法）到 0.953 不等（异物，数字方法）。几乎在所有的标准里，数字和传统方法的 ROC 曲线下的区域都无显著性差异。唯一例外的是集体标准中的纵隔异常，数字方法比传统方法有更好的结果（$P < 0.05$）。而在所有标准中除两个外（胸壁异常和钙化），数字系统等同或比传统系统略好一些，但无统计学意义。

答案

The area under the ROC curve depends on the different criteria and ranges from 0.687 (mediastinal abnormalities, conventional method) to 0.953 (foreign bodies, digital method). No significant differences were found between the area under the ROC curve of the digital and conventional methods for almost all criteria considered. The single exception was the collective criterion mediastinal abnormalities, for which the digital method gave better results than the conventional method ($P < 0.05$). However, in all criteria except two (chest wall abnormalities and calcifications), the digital system performed equally to or slightly better than the conventional system without being statistically significant.

chest wall 胸壁　　　foreign body 异物

第 149 天

学习

Overall image quality was ranked equal by at least five radiologists in 70% of cases. For the remaining images, overall image quality was judged significantly superior with the CRT display ($P < 0.001$). Agreement on equal display quality was reached by at least five of the seven radiologists for retrocardiac vessels in 85% of cases, for perihilar structures in 75% of cases, and for peripheral vessels in 74% of cases. For the contours of the trachea and for the lung parenchyma, the proportion of images with equal display quality was lower, at 51% and 54%, respectively. For the images judged differently, Wilcoxon's rank sum test found significant preferences ($P < 0.001$) for the CRT display in visualization of structures in low-attenuation areas of the thorax and for the LCD in visualization of structures in high-attenuation areas of the thorax. Delineation of the tracheal contour and retrocardiac vessels was ranked superiorly with LCD, whereas delineation of perihilar structures, peripheral vessels, and the lung parenchyma was ranked superiorly with CRT display.

至少有 5 位放射学家对 70% 的病例评判影像整体质量相同。对于其他影像，判定用 CRT 显示影像整体质量明显好（$P < 0.001$）。7 位放射学家中至少有 5 位对心后血管 85% 的病例显示质量意见一致，肺间结构 75%，外周血管 74%。对于气管轮廓、肺实质的病例意见一致较低，分别为 51%，54%。由于影像不同的判定方法，Wilcoxon 检验发现有显著倾向性（$P < 0.001$），胸部低衰减区结构是 CRT 显示占优，胸部高衰减结构 LCD 显示占优。对于气管轮廓和心后血管的显示用 LCD 具有优势，而对于肺门结构、外周血管和肺实质用 CRT 显示占优。

retrocardiac [ˌretrəu'kɑ:diæk] *a.* 心后的
perihilar [ˌperi'hailə] *a.* 肺门周围的
peripheral [pə'rifərəl] *a.* 外周的、周围的、末梢的
contour ['kɔntuə] *n.* 外形、轮廓
trachea ['treikiə] *n.* 气管
tracheal *a.* 气管的

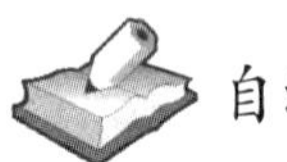
自测

心率水平和在绝对与相对时间间隔重建中 R-R 的起始点对图像质量的显著相关并未观察到（相对时间：r=0.23，P=0.79；绝对时间：r=0.31，P=0.62）。但是，通过聚类分析，我们找到图像质量最好的两个显著子群：在低心率时，最好的图像质量在舒张中期重建间隔；在高心率患者中，最好的图像质量在收缩末期和舒张早期重建间隔。同样，这些结果在基于相对和绝对时间重建图像中也可观察到。在心率较低时，相对时间平均起始点为 61% 的 R-R 间期（范围：40% ~ 75%），与之对应的是绝对时间重建中 R 后的 599.3 ms（范围：450 ~ 840 ms）；心率较高时，平均起始点分别为 27.3% 的 R-R 间期（范围：10% ~ 45%）和 R 后的 202.3 ms（范围：82 ~ 336 ms）。截止心率在收缩末期、舒张早期和舒张中期，从 64.0/min 到 68.5/min，并受检查血管和重建技术的影响（相对与绝对时间）。

答案

A significant correlation between the heart rate and the R-R starting points of the reconstruction intervals leading to best image quality was not observed for either reconstruction technique (relative timing, $r = 0.23$, $P = 0.79$; absolute timing, $r = 0.31$, $P = 0.62$). However, cluster analysis allowed us to identify two significant subgroups leading to best image quality: At low heart rates, best image quality was observed for middiastolic reconstruction intervals; at high heart rates, best image quality was observed for end-systolic and early-diastolic intervals. Likewise, these findings were observed for image reconstruction based on relative and absolute

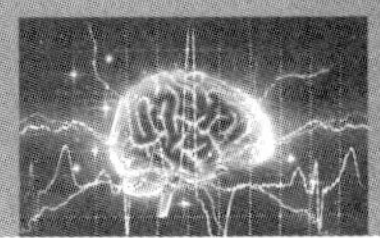

timing. At low heart rates, average starting points of the intervals were 61% of R-R interval (range, 40%—75%) in case of relative timing and 599.3 ms after R (range, 450—840 ms) in case of absolute timing; at high heart rates, average starting points were 27.3% of R-R interval (range, 10%—45%) and 202.3 ms after R (range, 82—336 ms). The cutoff heart rates for end-systolic, early-diastolic, and middiastolic image reconstruction ranged from 64.0 beats per minute to 68.5 beats per minute and were influenced by the vascular segment examined and the reconstruction technique used (relative vs absolute timing).

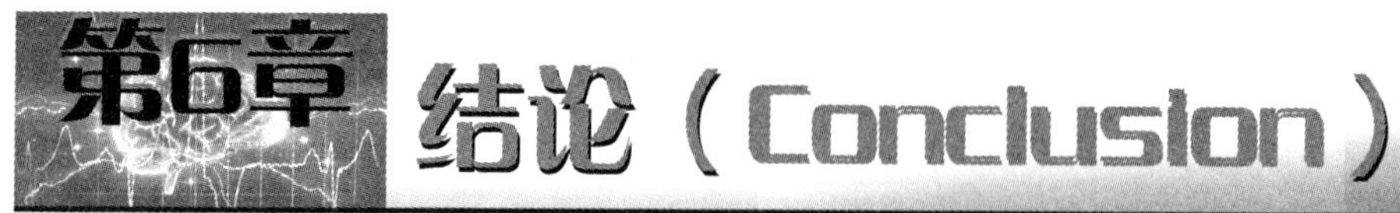

第6章 结论（Conclusion）

根据前面的结果言简意赅地推出相关的论断，是对作者该项研究成果的高度概括和总结。在此尤其要突出研究的普遍规律，画龙点睛地概述作者的学术观点，该项成果的最终价值；对于科研工作中的不足之处可一带而过。总之，结论应该建立在结果之上，应具有充分、真实、可靠的证据，并与前言、科研目的相呼应。

第 150 天

学习

In conclusion, this clinical study confirms that CsI/a-Si detector technology fully satisfies the requirements for chest radiography at a wall stand, even at a reduced detector dose.

总之，此临床研究证实 CsI/a-Si 探测器技术完全满足站立位胸部 X 线摄影需要，甚至可降低探测器剂量。

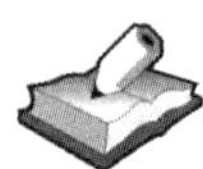

自测

总之，初步研究显示手、足硒数字 X 线摄影的主观影像质量与屏 - 片（速度为 100）成像质量相当。

答案

In conclusion, this initial study revealed that the subjective image quality of selenium-based digital radiographic images of the hand and foot is equivalent to that of film-screen images (100 speed).

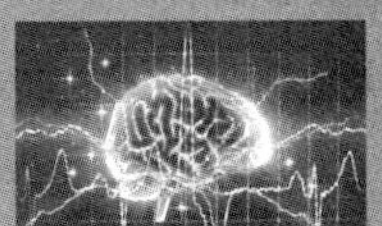

第 151 天

In conclusion, we describe a technique for direct coronal CT imaging that combines helical scanning with simplified patient positioning. This technique results in a rapid study with minimal patient-motion artifacts and has become the standard method for direct coronal wrist imaging in our institution.

总之,我们描述了一种直接冠状 CT 扫描技术,它将简单的患者定位与螺旋扫描相结合。此项技术可快速扫描以减少患者移动伪影,并已成为我所进行直接冠状腕部成像的标准方法。

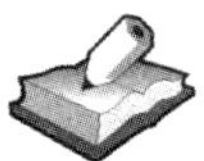

总之,单独应用组合螺旋 HRCT 胸部扫描的放射吸收剂量要比单独应用标准螺旋加轴位 HRCT 多 32%。因此,组合螺旋 HRCT 胸部扫描并不是一个可取的临床技术。

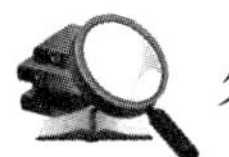

In conclusion, radiation absorbed dose is 32% greater in a single combination helical HRCT scan of the chest than the separate standard helical plus axial HRCT protocol. Combination helical HRCT scanning of the chest is, therefore, not a clinically advisable technique.

第 152 天

In this study, we proved that Xe ventilation CT with a DE technique was technically feasible for dynamic and static evaluation of regional ventilation. Xe ventilation CT with a DE technique yields a ventilation map and thin-section CT images.

在这项研究中,我们证实了使用双能量技术的 Xe 通气 CT 在动态和静态评价局部肺功能上的可行性。使用双能量技术的 Xe 通气 CT 给出了通气图和薄层的 CT 图像。

static ['stætik] *a.* 静止的,固定的

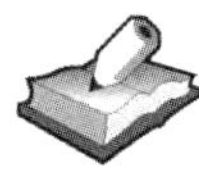

成像伪影会造成迷惑并会导致诊断上的不准确性。尽管在早期 CR 系统中出现的一些

伪影已得到解决，如当准直器不平行于暗盒边缘时引起的伪影，但是 CR 成像仍然还存在自己的一系列伪影。若把这些伪影与其他更多传统的成像模式相比，它们在 CR 成像中表现得完全不同。如果 CR 系统使用者们知道产生这些伪影的可能原因，那么有效地消除这些伪影将更容易。

答案

Imaging artefacts are distracting and can cause diagnostic inaccuracies. Although some of the artefacts found in early-generation CR systems have been addressed, such as those caused when collimation was not parallel to cassette edges, CR imaging continues to have its own set of artefacts. These artefacts can present differently on a CR image when compared with other more traditional modalities. If CR system users are aware of the probable causes of artefacts, it will be easier to efficiently eliminate them.

第 153 天

学习

The linear model is often defined as a conservative assumption. It is not conservative if we need a moderate dose rate of radiation to stimulate our immune system. Too little radiation appears to result in an earlier death. The analogy would be to reduce essential trace elements in our diet, because they are poisonous in large quantities.

线性体模常被认为是保守假设。如果我们需要适当的辐射剂量率刺激我们的免疫系统，那就不是一个保守的假设。罕见的辐射量会导致更早的死亡。相当于在我们的饮食中减少必需的微量元素，因为在大剂量情况下它们是有毒的。

conservative [kən'sə:vətiv] *a.* 保守的

assumption [ə'sʌmpʃən] *n.* 假设; make an assumption 假定; on the assumption that 假定

stimulate ['stimjuleit] *vt.* 刺激　　immune [i'mju:n] *a.* 免疫的

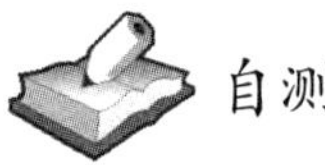
自测

CT 放射防护不应该变成主观遐想或臆断，但同时不能故步自封。患者和买主都有权利希望医护人员遵从最佳实践原则。就所涉及的医护人员和科室而言，这意味着要意识到不断涌现的资料及实践中潜在的变化，根据进展修正协定。同时也意味着建立当地剂量审查，以确保检查遵从已有的参考剂量水平，除非有临床正当理由才可超剂量。所有 CT 操作人员必须接受这一连续的过程。

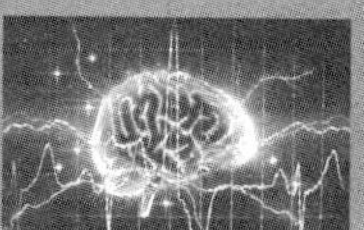

答案

Radiation protection in CT must not become subject to paranoia or a witch-hunt, but equally there is no place for complacency. Both patients and purchasers have the right to expect that staff conform to best practice principles. As far as staff and departments are concerned, this means an awareness of emerging evidence and the implied changes in practice, with revision of protocols to take account of advances. It also means establishing local dose audit to ensure that examinations conform to available reference dose levels except where there is clinical justification for exceeding these. This continuing process must be embraced by all who practice CT.

paranoia［ˌpærəˈnɔiə］*n.* 妄想狂、偏执狂

embrace［imˈbreis］*v.* 拥抱、接受

第 154 天

学习

We conclude from our data that, under ideal viewing conditions (subdued ambient lighting, no off-angle viewing) and without online windowing, the overall visibility of anatomic landmarks is equal with high-resolution CRT display and LCD for most images. If differences are appreciated, the LCD appears significantly superior for delineating structures in the mediastinum, and the CRT display appears significantly superior for delineating structures in the lung.

从我们的数据中得出结论，在理想的阅片条件下（周围光线柔和，没有斜视），不用在线调窗，采用高分辨率 CRT 显示与 LCD 显示对于大部分影像来讲解剖结构的整体能见度相同。如果考虑评估差异，纵隔结构的描绘 LCD 显示明显占优，而肺内结构的描述 CRT 显示明显占优。

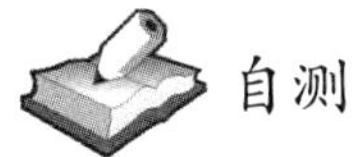
自测

总之，我们的研究中，对于诊断泌尿系结石，计算机 X 线摄影的软拷贝显示特性比硬拷贝影像好。此外，在 LCD 显示器上用软拷贝观察影像的诊断特性与在高分辨率图像显示器上观看软拷贝影像相似。这些结果表明在 PACS 环境中用软拷贝观看计算机 X 线照片应该使诊断特性类似于或略精确于激光打印胶片环境所得到的诊断特性。我们的结果也表明 LCD 显示器观看软拷贝影像有明显的临床可行性。

答案

In summary, in our study the soft-copy display of computed radiographs performed better than hard-copy images for detecting urinary calculi. In addition, the diagnostic performance with soft-copy images viewed on an LCD monitor was comparable to that of soft-copy images viewed on a high-resolution video monitor. These results suggest that computed radiographs viewed in a soft-copy PACS environment should result in diagnostic performance similar to or slightly more accurate than that obtained in a laser-printed film-based environment. Our results also suggest the distinct clinical feasibility of the LCD monitor for viewing soft-copy images.

第 155 天

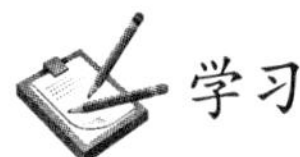
学习

We conclude that the diagnostic performance of the new large-area silicon flat-panel detector is equivalent or superior to that of the conventional screen-film system in clinical chest imaging and can replace conventional radiographic system. This new technology offers the transmission and storage possibilities inherent to digital radiology, which could facilitate daily practice and reduce the initial high costs in the long-term.

我们的结论：这种新型大面积硅平板探测器的诊断性能在临床胸部成像中等同于或优于传统屏 - 片系统，并可取代传统 X 线照相系统。这项新技术具有数字影像特有的传输、存储的能力，这使每天工作简便，随着时间的推移可降低最初的高成本。

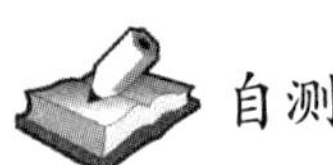
自测

总之，用基于 a-Si 的平板探测器所获得的影像质量和结构的显示能力等同于或优于传统屏 - 片 X 线摄影系统所获得的影像。尽管数字 X 线照片的放射剂量比屏 - 片 X 线照片大约降低 50%，但此发现是可靠的。进一步临床研究是期望比较平板探测器系统与传统屏 - 片系统的诊断精确性。

答案

In conclusion, the image quality and the visibility of structures on the images obtained with a flat-panel detector based on amorphous silicon were perceived as equal or superior to images obtained with a conventional film-screen radiography system. This finding was true even though the radiation dose of the digital radiographs was reduced approximately 50% compared with the film-screen radiographs. Further clinical studies are desirable to compare the diagnostic accuracy of the flat-panel detector system to that of conventional film-screen system.

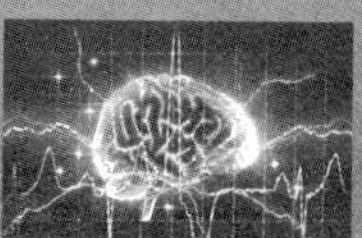

第 156 天

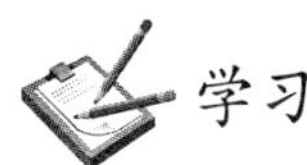

学习

In summary, for large corporations, a fixed facility can be a successful means of providing breast cancer screening to employees and their dependents. High-quality mammography services that are well accepted by beneficiaries can be provided at a reasonable cost. In addition to producing health care cost savings associated with early detection, such programs engender feelings of goodwill toward the company among its workforce.

总之,对于大公司,一个固定装置对雇员及其家属进行乳腺癌普查是一个成功的方法。受益者很乐意接受这样既经济、质量又高的乳腺 X 线影像服务。它不仅节约早期诊断保健费用,这样的健康项目还使雇员对公司产生友好的感情。

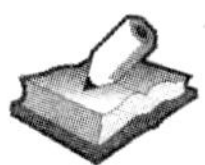

自测

尽管差异无统计学意义,但在整个病变的诊断方面具有约 11 lp/mm 空间分辨率的数字乳腺 X 线摄影略优于 16 lp/mm 空间分辨率的传统乳腺 X 线摄影。数字乳腺 X 线摄影的对比灵敏度的增强弥补了它的低空间分辨率。因此,不需要在各个方面匹配胶片就可以达到屏 - 片系统的诊断精确性。

答案

Digital spot mammography with a spatial resolution of about 11 lp/mm was slightly superior in overall lesion detection to conventional spot mammography with a spatial resolution of about 16 lp/mm, although the difference was not statistically significant. The enhanced contrast sensitivity of digital mammography could compensate for its lower spatial resolution. Therefore, to achieve diagnostic accuracy equal to that of film, it is not necessary to match the film in all respects.

compensate ['kɔmpenseit] *v.* 补偿

第 157 天

学习

In summary, we found that failures in positioning were associated with subsequent interval cancer occurrence under all conditions considered. Failures in the measures of sharpness were associated with interval cancer occurrence depending on the cancers included; follow-up periods;

and adjustments for age, year of study, and breast density. Our results emphasize the importance of attention to positioning and indicate that accepting even borderline positioning that reduces the visualization of the pectoralis muscle or the nipple may increase the likelihood of missing an invasive breast cancer and reduce the sensitivity of mammography.

总之,在所有考虑到的条件下我们发现定位失败与间隔癌的发生有关。锐利度测试的失败与间隔癌的产生有关,取决于所涉及的癌症复查期间、随访时间以及对年龄、检查时间、乳腺密度的调整。我们的结果强调注意定位的重要性,并指出接受减少胸肌或乳头显示的边缘定位可增加有创乳腺癌的漏诊,并降低乳腺 X 线摄影的灵敏度。

pectoralis [ˌpektəˈreilis] *a.* 胸的

nipple [ˈnipl] *n.* 乳头

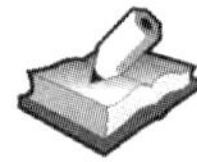
自测

在乳腺 X 线照片中,适当地保证临床影像质量比放射学的任何其他领域更具有挑战。在乳腺 X 线摄影中,适当的临床影像质量不仅需要先进的设备,而且需要在医学物理师的监督下全面地、频繁地校准及质量控制。乳腺定位、压迫及技术选择的技巧是一门科学艺术。技术员细心、一致、谨慎地应用 3 项技巧是同等关键的。当放射学家判读每 1 次检查时,他或她也将评价临床影像质量,以反馈给医学物理师及技术专家。

答案

Maintenance of proper clinical image quality in mammography represents a greater challenge than in any other area of radiology. In mammography, proper clinical image quality requires not only state-of-the-art equipment but also extensive and frequent calibration and quality control under the supervision of a medical physicist. The skills of breast positioning, compression, and technique selection are an art based on science. Careful, consistent, conscientious application of these skills by the technologist is equally critical. As the radiologist interprets each examination, he or she should also evaluate clinical image quality to provide feedback to the medical physicist and technologist.

第 158 天

学习

In conclusion, our results indicate that in 16-row detector cardiac CT, image quality critically depends on the choice of a suited reconstruction interval and reconstruction technique. In patients with a high heart rate, the best image quality is observed in end systole and early diastole;

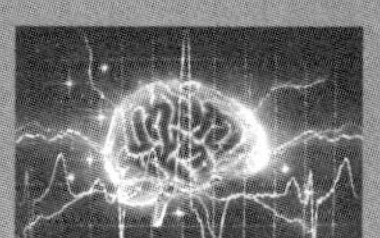

in patients with a lower heart rate, the best image quality is observed in mid-diastole. Image reconstruction based on absolute timing leads to significantly better image quality, but it does not significantly increase diagnostic accuracy compared with that achieved by using relative timing. Although best image quality is always obtained in patients with a low heart rate, the choice of a suitable reconstruction interval may allow sufficient image quality in patients with a high heart rate.

总之，我们的研究结果表明，在 16 排探测器 CT 中，心脏断层图像质量的关键在于选择一种适合的重建间隔及重建技术。观察高心率患者最佳的图像质量在收缩末期及舒张早期；观察低心率患者最佳的图像质量在舒张中期。基于绝对时间的图像重建有更好的图像质量，但并不比相对时间重建可显著提高诊断准确率。虽然最佳的图像质量经常在低心率患者中获得，但在高心率患者中选择一种合适的重建间隔可以保证有良好的图像质量。

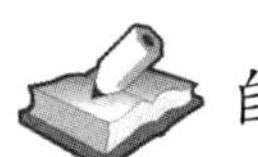

自测

总的来说，我们证明了双源 CT 通过改善时间分辨率为图像质量提供了一个较广的心率范围，使图像质量从心率的限制中独立出来。然而检查期间的心率变化对图像质量有普遍的影响，对于图像质量有一个很大的下降，然而不会对诊断的正确率产生明显的下降。这个发现对于那些接受 β 受体阻滞药或者原来由于心律失常而不能接受检查的患者有重要的影响，而且最终可能会放宽能进行冠状动脉 CT 成像的临床指针。随着将来时间分辨率的进一步提高，钙化会成为降低图像质量的最根本的因素，而且会成为正确诊断的主要挑战。

答案

In conclusion, we demonstrated that improved temporal resolution with dual-source CT provided heart-rate independent image quality within a wide range of patient heart rates. While interexamination variability has a persistent impact on global image quality, there is a large cutoff for good image quality and no translation of effect on the deterioration of accuracy. Such findings have important implications for the administration of beta-blockers or exclusion of patients with arrhythmia and may eventually broaden the clinical indications for coronary CT angiography. With further increase of temporal resolution, calcification emerges as the primary cause of degrading image quality and continues to pose a fundamental challenge to diagnostic accuracy.

第 159 天

学习

In conclusion, our results indicate that this digital subtraction technique for chest radiographs can provide improved accuracy for detection of subtle new abnormalities greater than 1 cm in diameter when paired digitized previous and current chest radiographs are viewed in conjunction with the temporal subtraction images. Findings in the observer test showed a remarkable increase in both sensitivity and specificity, with the additional benefit of a reduction in mean reading time. These results were obtained with a selected set of cases and are therefore of a preliminary nature. This design was necessary to keep the observer test to a manageable size. Additional studies in a prospective clinical setting will be needed to further validate this technique, specifically with regard to its diagnostic value in opacities with other origins and sizes. This method could be readily implemented on a digital workstation, with previous images from a digital archive being automatically registered and subtracted prior to interpretation. Potential clinical applications include lung cancer screening, follow-up of patients with thoracic neoplasms, and monitoring of patients at risk for opportunistic infections.

结论：通过观察配对数字化先前和当前胸部X线照片以及即时减影图像时，我们的结果证明此项数字减影技术对于胸部X线照片能改善直径大于 1 cm 的新的异常诊断精度。在观察者测试中发现，灵敏度和特异性显著增加，附加的好处是平均判读时间减少。由于是从选择的这组病例获取这些结果，因此，这也是必然的。此项设计需要使观察者测试在易控制范围内。今后需要在临床上进一步确认这项技术，特别考虑它在阴影的位置和大小方面的诊断价值。这个方法能在数字工作站中快速执行，使来自数字文档的先前影像自动影像匹配且在判读前减影。潜在的临床应用包括肺癌的普查，胸部肿瘤患者的随访，并对有传染机会的危险患者实行监控。

neoplasm ['ni(:)əuplæzəm] *n.* 新生物、肿瘤

validate ['vælideit] *vt.* 确认、证实

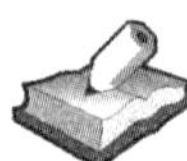
自测

总而言之，没有科学证据证明低剂量照射没有风险，即使乐观来看也是没有定论的。政策上的考虑并不能给出一个基于低剂量阈值的制度，那会导致照射剂量的增加和与之相伴的风险的加大。此外，要说服公众的普遍看法去放宽放射性的利用限制也是很难的，这将会遭受媒体和环保社团的强烈批评，进而丧失公众的信任。实践中执行一个阈值模型也是相当困难的，因为没有简单的方法去评价风险。风险效益评估的基础将会更改，它目前正运用在证明研究计划、规划放射设施、限制放射物质排放以及争论所有运用辐射的实践中，但是并没有任何清晰的可以替代的方法被提出来。用 LNT 办法实施辐射防护遭到摒弃的时机尚未来临，同样在医疗保健或其他利用电离辐射的活动也不会很快结束。

答案

In conclusion, the scientific evidence does not show that there is no risk from radiation at low

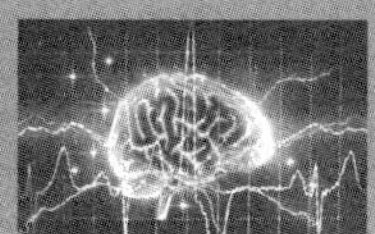

doses. It is at best inconclusive. Political justification cannot be given to a system based on a low dose threshold that could lead to increased exposures with greater associated risk. Moreover, it would be hard to convince the public of the wisdom for relaxing controls on the use of radiation, and this would be likely to lead to heavy criticism from the press and the environmental lobby, leading to loss of public confidence. Practical implementation of a threshold model would be more difficult because there would be no simple method with which to assess risk. The basis for risk benefit assessments carried out currently in justifying research proposals, planning radiation facilities, restricting radioactive discharges and justifying all practices using radiation would be removed, without any clear alternative methodology being provided in its place. The time is not yet nigh when the LNT approach to implementation of radiation protection should be abandoned, either in healthcare or in other practices using ionizing radiation.

methodology [meθəˈdɔlədʒi] *n.* 方法

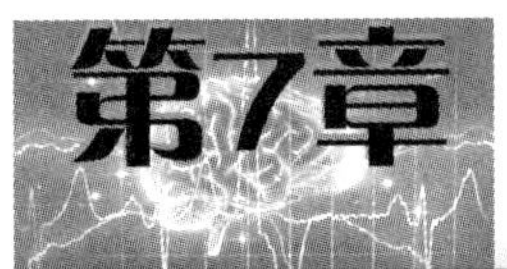

第7章 致谢（Acknowledgments）

致谢主要是用来感谢非直接参与科研工作的人们所给予作者的支持、帮助，以及资助等，最常用的句型是 thank…for…。

第 160 天

学习

1. We thank the technicians in our department for their help.
   感谢我们科的技术员所给予的帮助。
2. Special thanks to Zhang San and Li Si for their help.
   特别感谢张三和李四的帮助。

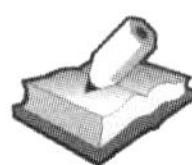

自测

1. 我们感谢张三和李四为研究的实际判断及其领悟所付出的努力。
2. 我们衷心感谢合作医院儿科和放射科同仁们的合作。

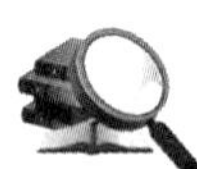

答案

1. We thank Zhang San and Li Si for their efforts regarding the practical part and realization of the study.
2. We gratefully acknowledge the cooperation of the staff at paediatric and radiation physics units at the participating hospitals.

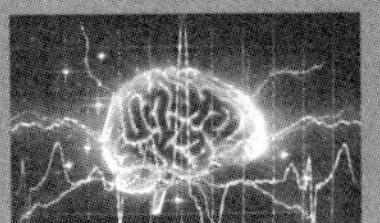

第 161 天

学习

We thank Dr.Wang for providing us with Figure 1.
我们感谢王博士为我们提供图 1 照片。

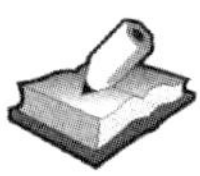

自测

1. 我们感谢王博士所进行的放射剂量测试。
2. 我们感谢王博士对我们研究中所作的统计学贡献。

答案

1. We thank Dr. Wang for performing the radiation dose measurements.
2. We thank Dr. wang for expert statistical contributions to our study.

附录 A

词汇表(Glossary)

A

a wide dynamic range 宽的动态范围

abdomen['æbdəmen, æb'dəumen]n. 腹部

abdominal[æb'dɔminl]a. 腹部的

abnormal[æb'nɔ:ml]a. 异常的

absolute tachyarrhythmia 绝对性心律失常

acquisition time 采集时间

acquisition[ækwi'ziʃən]n. 获取、采集

acrylic[ə'krilik]a. 丙烯酸的、聚丙烯

actual['æktjuəl]a. 实际的、事实上

acute abdomen 急腹症

acute coronary syndrome 急性冠状动脉综合征

acute[ə'kju:t]a. 急性的

adjacent[ə'dʒeisənt]n. 邻近的、毗连的

administer[əd'ministə]vt. 给予、用药

adult['ædʌlt]a. 成人的, n. 成人

advantage[əd'vɑ:ntidʒ]n. 优势、有利条件

agent['eidʒənt]n. 剂

thick section 厚层

algorithm['ælgəriðəm]n. 算法、规则系统

allergic[ə'lə:dʒik]a. 过敏性的、变应性的

alter['ɔ:ltə]v. 改变、变更

ambient['æmbiənt]a. 周围的、环境的

amorphous silicon 非晶硅

amperage['æmpəridʒ]n. 安培数、电流量、电流强度

an antiscatter grid 防散射滤线栅

an erect position 立位

analog-to-digital converter 模数转换器,简称 ADC

anatomic landmark 解剖标志

anatomic structures 解剖结构

anatomy[ə'nætəmi]n. 解剖学、解剖

aneurysm['ænjuərizəm]n. 动脉瘤

angle['æŋgl]n. 角度

angulation[æŋgju'leiʃən]n. 角度

annotate['ænəteit]v. 注释、注解

antecubital['ænti'kjubitəl]a. 肘前的

anthropomorphic a. 拟人的、类人的

antireflective a. 抗反射的

aorta[ei'ɔ:tə]n. 主动脉; 复数 aortae[ei'ɔ:ti:]或 aortas

approximately[ə'prɔksimitli]ad. 近似地、大致

array[ə'rei]n. 排、列

arterial[ɑ:'tiəriəl]a. 动脉的

arthritis[ɑ:'θraitis]n. 关节炎; 复数 arthritides[ɑ:'θritidi:z]

arthroscopy[ɑ:'θrɔskəpi]n. 关节镜检查

artifact['ɑ:tifækt] = artefact n. 伪影

ascending aorta 升主动脉

ascertain[æsə'tein]vt. 确定、查明

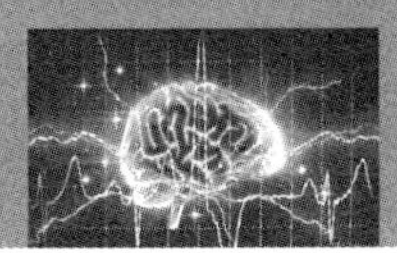

aspect ['æspekt] n.(问题、事物等的)方面
aspiration ['æspə'reiʃən] n. 吸引术、抽吸
assist in doing sth.(或 assist sb. with sth.,或 assist to do sth.)有助于
assumption [ə'sʌmpʃən] n. 假设
asymmetric [æsi'metrik] a. 不对称、不平衡
asymptomatic [ˌeisimptə'mætik] a. 无症状的
at a soft-copy viewing workstation 软拷贝观察工作站
at random 任意、随取
atelectasis [ˌætə'lektəsis] n. 肺不张
atherosclerosis n. 粥样硬化
attending physician 主治医师
attenuation [ətenju'eiʃən] n. 衰减
auditory ['ɔ:ditəri] a. 听的、听觉的
automatic exposure control 自动曝光控制
avascular [ə'væskjulə] a. 无血管的
axial ['æksiəl] a. 轴的,轴向的

B

basal thyroid-stimulating hormone 基础促甲状腺激素
be derived from 从……产生的
be known to 为……所知
be relevant to(with)和……有关的
be scheduled to 预备做某事
be similar to 与……相似
be submitted to 送请、已提交
be superior in 在……方面占优势, be superior to 优于、胜过
be superior to M in N 在 N 方面比 M 好
be unaware of 不知情
benign [bi'nain] a. 良性的
beta-blocker β 受体阻滞药
bias ['baiəs] n. 偏见、倾向性、癖好
bilateral [bai'lætərəl] a. 两侧的
binomial [bai'nəumiəl] n. 二项式
biopsy ['baiɔpsi] n,vt. 活检
bladder ['blædə] n. 膀胱
blooming ['blu:miŋ] n. 模糊现象、开花效应
blur [blə:] v. 变模糊
bolus triggering technique 团注激发技术
bolus ['bəuləs] n. 团、块
bone window 骨窗
bony ['bəuni] a. 骨的
border ['bɔ:də] n. 边缘、边界
brain [brein] n. 脑
breast phantom 乳腺体模
breast [brest] n. 乳房、乳腺
bronchus ['brɔŋkəs] n. 支气管; 复数 bronchi ['brɔŋkai]
bulk [bʌlk] n. 大量、容量
bulky ['bʌlki] a. 体积大的、笨重的
burden ['bə:dn] n. 负担

C

calcification ['kælsifi'keiʃən] n. 钙化
calculus ['kælkjuləs](复 数 calculuses 或 calculi)n. 结石
calyceal ['kæli'siəl] a. 盏的
cancer ['kænsə] n. 癌、癌症、恶性肿瘤
cancer in situ 原位癌
candela [kæn'delə] n. 堪德拉(发光强度单位)
canthus ['kænθəs] n. 眦,眼角; 复数 canthi ['kænθai]
capsule ['kæpsju:l] n. 小盒、容器
capture ['kæptʃə] n./vt. 捕捉、收集
carbon ['kɑ:bən] n. 碳
cardiac cycle 心脏周期
cardiac failure 心脏衰竭

cardiac imaging 心脏成像
cardiac software package 心脏软件包
carpal ['kɑ:pl] *a.* 腕的
cassette [kæ'set] *n.* 暗盒
catheter ['kæθitə] *n.* 导管
cathode ray tube 阴极射线管，简称 CRT
cesium iodide 碘化铯
challenge ['tʃælindʒ] *n.* 挑战
characteristic [ˌkæriktə'ristik] *n.* 特征、性能
charge-coupled device 电子耦合器件，简称 CCD
chaser ['tʃeisə] *n.* 追逐者
chest radiographs 胸部 X 线照片
chest [tʃest] *n.* 胸、胸廓
chest wall 胸壁
chief physician 主任医师
circular ['sə:kjulə] *a.* 圆形的、环状的、循环的
cirrhosis [si'rəusis] *n.* 硬变
classification [ˌklæsifi'keiʃən] *n.* 分类
clinical ['klinikəl] *a.* 临床的、临床上的
cluster ['klʌstə] *v.* 成群、群集、簇集
cohort ['kəuhɔ:t] *n.* 一群
collimation [kɔli'meiʃən] *n.* 准直
collimator ['kɔlimeitə] *n.* 准直器
commercially available 用于商业用途
committee [kə'miti] *n.* 委员会
community hospital 社区医院
comparative [kəm'pærətiv] *a.* 比较的
compatible [kəm'pætəbl] *a.* 相容的
compensate ['kɔmpenseit] *v.* 补偿
complex ['kɔmpleks] *a.* 复杂的
complication [ˌkɔmpli'keiʃən] *n.* 并发症
composition [kɔmpə'ziʃən] *n.* 组成、成分、构成、合成
compression [kəm'preʃən] *n.* 压缩、加压、压力
computed radiography 计算机 X 线摄影，简称 CR
computed tomography 计算机断层扫描，简称 CT
computer hardware and software 计算机硬软件
concordance [kən'kɔ:dəns] *n.* 一致、协调
confidence level 可信度
consecutive [kən'sekjutiv] *a.* 连续的
consensus [kən'sensəs] *n.*（意见）一致，同意
consent [kən'sent] *v.* 同意
conservative [kən'sə:vətiv] *a.* 保守的
conspicuity *n.* 能见度
conspicuous [kən'spikjuəs] *a.* 显著的、明显的
consumer-oriented 面向消费者的
contour ['kɔntuə] *n.* 外形、轮廓
contrast resolution 对比分辨率
contrast-enhanced 对比增强
contribute to　产生
control study 对照研究
control [kən'trəul] *v.* 控制、管理
conventional film-screen radiography 传统屏 - 片 X 线摄影
conventional hard-copy imaging 传统硬拷贝成像
conventional radiography 传统 X 线摄影
convert M to(into) N　把 M 转变成 N
converter *n.* 转换器
convolution [kɔnvə'lu:ʃən] *n.* 卷积
coordinate [kəu'ɔ:dinit] *n.* 坐标系
corneal *a.* 角膜的
coronal [kə'rəunəl] *a.* 冠状的
coronary angiography 冠状动脉血管造影
coronary artery stenosis 冠状动脉狭窄
coronary artery stent 冠状动脉扩张
corresponding *a.* 相当的、对应的、一致的
cortical ['kɔ:tikəl] *a.* 皮质
counterpart ['kauntəpɑ:t] *n.* 一对中之一
couple ['kʌpl] *vt.* 连接、结合、使耦合
coverage ['kʌvəridʒ] *n.* 覆盖

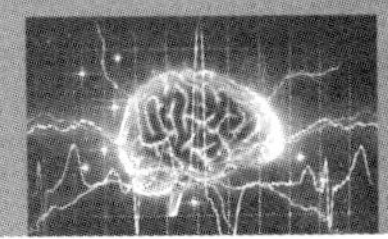

crosshair ['krɔ:shεə] *n.* 十字准线
cross-sectional image 横断面影像
CT dose index CT 剂量指数
current ['kʌrənt] *a.* 当前的
curved-planar reformation 曲面重组
cyclotron ['saikləutrɔn] *n.* 回旋加速器
cylindrical [sə'lindrikl] *a.* 圆柱的、圆筒形的

D

defect [di'fekt] *n.* 缺损、缺陷
delineation [dilini'eiʃn] *n.* 轮廓、描绘
detective quantum efficiency 量子检出效率，简称 DQE
detector-focus distance 探测器与焦点之间的距离
development [di'veləpmənt] *n.* 显影、冲洗
device [di'vais] *n.* 装置、设备、器件
devise [di'vaiz] *v.* 设计、创造、产生
diagnostic [ˌdaiəg'nɔstik] *a.* 诊断的
diameter [dai'æmitə] *n.* 直径
diaphragm ['daiəfræm] *n.* 膈
diastole [dai'æstəli] *n.* 舒张期
diatrizoate meglumine 泛影葡胺
digital imaging and communications in medicine 医学数字成像与传输，简称 DICOM
digital radiography 数字 X 线摄影，简称 DR
digital subtraction angiography 数字减影血管造影
dim [dim] (dimmed; dimming) *v.* 变暗淡，dim out 遮暗
diminish [di'miniʃ] *v.* 减少、缩小、递减、削弱
direct-readout radiography system 直接判读 X 线摄影系统
discrepancy [dis'krepəsi] *n.* 不同、差异
discrete [dis'kri:t] *a.* 分离的、分散的、稀疏的
disease [di'zi:z] *n.* 疾病
display [dis'plei] *vt.* 显示、呈现
dissipate ['disipeit] *v.* 消散、消除
distortion [di'stɔ:ʃn] *n.* 变形、失真
divergent [dai'və:dʒənt] *a.* 发散的、辐射状的
dosage ['dəusidʒ] *n.* 剂量
dose [dəus] *n.* 剂量
dosimeter [dəu'simitə] *n.* 剂量仪
double-echo steady-state 双回波稳态
dual-energy technique 双能量技术
dual-segment reconstruction algorithms 双扇区重建算法
dual-source CT 双源 CT
duct [dʌkt] *n.* 导管
duration [djuə'reiʃən] *n.* 持续
dynamic range 动态范围

E

echo time 回波时间
echo train length 回波链长度
edge enhancement 边缘增强
effect [i'fekt] *n.* 作用、效应、影响
effective section thickness 有效层厚
efficacious [efi'keiʃəs] *a.* 有效的
effusion [i'fju:ʒən] *n.* 渗出、渗出液
either…or… 或者……或者，不论……还是
electric charge 电子电荷
electron-beam CT 电子束 CT
elevated ['eliveitid] *a.* 升高的
eligible ['elidʒəbl] *a.* 符合被推选条件的
eliminate [i'limineit] *vt.* 消除
embrace [im'breis] *v.* 拥抱、接受
emerge [i'mə:dʒ] *vi.* 浮现、出现、形成
emergency [i'mə:dʒənsi] *n.* 急症
emergent [i'mə:dʒənt] *a.* 紧急的、意外的

emission[i'miʃn]*n.* 发射
enhance[in'hɑ:ns]*vt.* 增强
environment[in'vaiərənmənt]*n.* 周围环境
equip[i'kwip]*vt.* 装备(equipped, equipping)
equivalent[i'kwivələnt]*a.* 相同的、相当的、等价的、等效的
establish[is'tæbliʃ]*vt.* 建立、形成、产生、证实
ethics['eθiks]*n.* 伦理
evacuate[i'vækjueit]*vt.* 排空
excision[ik'siʒn]*n.* 切除
excretory[iks'kri:təri]*a.* 排泄的
exist[ig'zist]*vi.* 存在、有
expectancy[ik'spektənsi]*n.* 预期、期望
expiration[ˌekspə'reiʃn]*n.* 呼出
exploit[ik'splɔit]*vt.* 开发、利用
exposure[ik'spəuʒə]*n.* 曝光、照射
exquisite[ik'skwizit]*a.* 灵敏的
external[ik'stə:nl]*a.* 外的、外部的
extinction *n.* 衰减
extraneous[ik'streiniəs]*a.* 外部的
extremity[ik'streməti]末端,肢

F

faceplate['feispleit]*n.* 荧光屏
facility[fə'siliti]*n.* 容易、方便、灵活、装置(常为复数)
factor['fæktə]*n.* 因素、原因
fast low-angle shot sequence 快速小角度激发脉冲序列
fast[fɑ:st]*vi.* 禁食
fat-suppression technique 脂肪抑制技术
feasible['fi:zəbl]*a.* 可行的
feedback['fi:dbæk]*n.* 反馈
fibre['faibə]*n.* 纤维
field of view 显示野(扫描野)
file[fail]*n.* 文件、档案
film-focus distance 焦 - 片距,也称 FFD
film-screen combination 屏 - 片组合
financial[fai'nænʃəl]*a.* 财政上的,财务的
fixed[fikst]*a.* 固定的
flat-panel detector 平板探测器
flat-panel digital radiography system 平板数字 X 线摄影系统
flat-panel display 平面显示器
flat-panel X-ray detector 平板 X 线探测器
flexibility[ˌfleksə'biləti]*n.* 灵活性、机动性
flip angle 翻转角
flow rate 流率
fluorescent screen 荧光屏、荧光板
flying focal spot technique 飞焦点技术
focal['fəukl]*a.* 焦点的
focal spot size 焦点大小
follow-up['fɔləu'ʌp]*n.* 随访
foot-lambert 英尺朗伯(亮度单位)
foreign body 异物
fracture['fræktʃə]*n.* 骨折
frame[freim]*n.* 框架
frontal['frʌntl]*n.* 正面、前面
full-field direct digital mammography 全视野直接数字乳腺 X 线摄影
functional['fʌŋkʃənl]*a.* 功能的、函数的

G

gadopentetate dimeglumine[ˌgædə'pentəteit daiˌmeglumi:n]钆喷酸二甲基葡胺
gantry rotation speed 机架旋转速度
generation[dʒenə'reiʃən]*n.* 产生、引起
generator['dʒenəreitə]*n.* 发生器
geometry[dʒi'ɔmətri]*n.* 几何学
gold standard 金标准

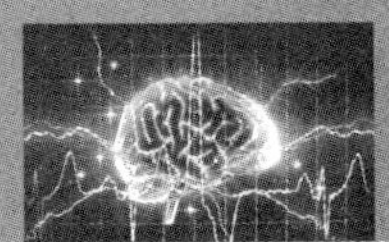

gradient echo 梯度回波
gradient-switch 梯度开关
gray-scale 灰阶
grid 滤线栅
guide [gaid] *vt.* 引导
handling *n.* 操作

H

hard-copy 硬拷贝
heal [hi:l] *v.* 治愈
helical ['helikl] *a.* 螺旋的
Helsinki ['helsiŋki] *n.* 赫尔辛基(芬兰首都)
high kilovoltage 高千伏
high optical densities 高光学密度
high-resolution CT 高分辨率 CT,简称 HRCT
high-voltage generator 高压发生器
hilum *n.* 门
hypersensitivity [ˌhaipə(:)'sensə'tivəti] *n.* 过敏反应、超敏反应
hyperthyroidism [ˌhaipə(:)'θairɔidizəm] *n.* 甲状腺功能亢进症

I

identify [ai'dentifai] *v.* 识别、辨认
illustrate ['iləstreit] *v.* 图解、举例说明
image quality 影像质量
imaging plate 成像板,简称 IP
immune [i'mju:n] *a.* 免疫的
impediment [im'pedimənt] *n.* 阻碍、障碍
a major impediment to ……的主要障碍
implement ['impliment] *n.* 器械、仪器
in a similar way to 与……相似的方式
in addition to 除……之外
in particular 特别是、尤其是
incident ['insidənt] *a.* 入射的
incorporate [in'kɔ:pəreit] *v.* 插入
increment ['inkrəmənt] *n.* 增量、递增
individual circulation time 个体循环时间
induce [in'dju:s] *vt.* 诱发、引起、导致
inferior [in'fiəriə] *a.* 下方的
inhomogeneity ['inˌhəumədʒi'ni:iti] *n.* 不均匀性
initiation [iˌniʃi'eiʃən] *n.* 开始
initiative [i'niʃətiv] *a.* 初步的
inspiration [ˌinspə'reiʃən] *n.* 吸气
institution [ˌinsti'tju:ʃn] *n.* 学校、研究所
instruct [in'strʌkt] *vt.* 讲授、说明
integrate ['intigreit] *vt.* 使结合; *vi.*(与……)结合起来(with)
intensifying screen 增感屏
intensity [in'tensiti] *n.* 强度
interlace [intə'leis] *n.* 间隔
intersection gap 层间距
interstitium [intəs'tiʃəm] *n.* 间质组织
interval ['intəvl] *n.* 间隔、间期
intracranial [ˌintrə'kreiniəl] *a.* 颅内的
intravenous injection 静脉注射
intravenous urography 静脉尿路造影术
invasive coronary angiography 有创冠状动脉血管造影
iodinated contrast media 碘对比剂
iohexol ['aiəu'heksɔl] *n.* 碘海醇
ionizing radiation 电离辐射
irradiation [ireidi'eiʃən] *n.* 照射、辐射
irregular heartbeat 不规则心率
isolate ['aisəleit] *vt.* 隔绝
isotropic [ˌaisə'trɔpik] *a.* 各向同性的
It is concluded that... 结论是……
It is estimated that... 估计……
It is recommended that... 建议……
It is suggested that... 建议……

It was found that… 发现……

It was observed that… 观察到……

J

joint [dʒɔint] *n.* 关节

junior ['dʒu:njə] *n.* 年少者

justify ['dʒʌstifai] *vt.* 证明为正当，为……辩护

L

lambert ['læmbə:t] *n.* 朗伯（亮度单位，物体表面垂直方向上每平方厘米反射或辐射一“流明”的亮度）

larger dynamic range 较大的动态范围

laser film 激光胶片

laser imager 激光相机

laser ['leizə] *n.* 激光

laser-printed 激光打印

lateral ['lætərəl] *a.* 侧的

lesion ['li:ʒn] *n.* 损害、损伤

lethal ['li:θl] *a.* 致死的

limited ['limitid] *a.* 有限的

line pairs per millimetre 每毫米线对（lp/mm）

linear ['liniə] *a.* 线型的，线的

liquid crystal display 液晶显示，简称 LCD

localization [ˌləukəlai'zeiʃn] *n.* 定位、局限

longevity [lɔn'dʒevəti] *n.* 长寿

loss [lɔs,lɔ:s] *n.* 丢失、损失；loss of 损失

low optical densities 低光学密度

low-cost 低成本的

low-noise receptor 低噪声接收器

lumbar ['lʌmbə] *a.* 腰的

lumen ['lu:men] *n.* 腔；复数 lumens 或 lumina ['lu:minə]

luminal ['lju:minæl] *a.* 腔的

luminance ['lu:minəns] *n.* 亮度

lung [lʌŋ] *n.* 肺

lung window 肺窗

M

magnetic resonance imaging 磁共振成像，简称 MRI

magnification [ˌmægnifi'keiʃn] *n.* 放大、放大率、放大倍数

magnify ['mægnifai] *vt.* 放大

main pulmonary artery 主肺动脉

majority [mə'dʒɔriti] *n.* 大部分

make an assumption 假定

malignant [mə'lignənt] *a.* 恶性的

mammography [mæ'mɔgrəfi] *n.* 乳腺 X 线摄影

manipulate [mə'nipjuleit] *v.* 操作、控制

Mann-Whitney test 两个独立样本的非参数检验，用于对两总体分布的比较判断

manufacturer [ˌmænju'fæktʃərə] *n.* 厂商

margin ['mɑ:dʒin] *n.* 边缘

mass [mæs] *n.* 肿块

marker ['mɑ:kə] *n.* 标记

matrix ['meitriks]（复数 matrices 或 matrixes）*n.* 基质、矩阵

matrix size 矩阵大小

maximum intensity projection 最大密度投影，简称 MIP

meatus [mi'eitəs] *n.* 道；复数 meatus（es）

mechanism ['mekənizəm] *n.* 机械、装置

mediastinal [ˌmi:diæs'tainəl] *a.* 纵隔的

mediastinal window 纵隔窗

mediastinum [ˌmi:diæs'tainəm] *n.* 纵隔；复数 mediastina [ˌmi:diæs'tainə]

medical ['medikəl] *a.* 医学的、医疗的、内科的

medicine ['medisin] *n.* 医学

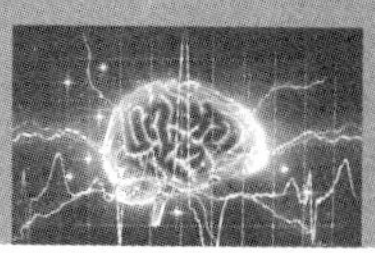

meniscal ['məniskl] a. 半月板的
metatarsal [ˌmetə'tɑ:sl] n. 跖骨
method ['meθəd] n. 方法
methodology [meθə'dɔlədʒi] n. 方法
milliampere-second 毫安秒
misregistration n. 配准不良、位置不正
modality [məu'dæləti] n. 模态、方式
moderate ['mɔdərət] a. 适度的、有节制的
module ['mɔdju:l] n. 模件
monitor ['mɔnitə] n. 显示器
monochrome ['mɔnəkrəum] n. 黑白图像
monophasic [mɔnə'feizik] a. 单相的
morphologic ['mɔ:fə'lɔdʒik] n. 形态学
mortality [mɔ:'tæliti] n. 致命性、死亡率
motion ['məuʃn] n. 运动、移位
motion artifact 移动伪影
motionless ['məuʃnləs] a. 不动的、固定的、静止的
mount [maunt] v. 安装
mount up 安装
moving and stationary grids 移动或固定滤线栅
moving grid 活动滤线栅
MR imaging 磁共振成像
mucosal a. 黏膜
multi-detector row spiral CT 多排探测器螺旋 CT
multiplanar reformation 多平面重组,简称 MPR
musculoskeletal [ˌmʌskjuləu'skelətəl] a. 肌与骨骼的
myelography [ˌmai'lɔgrəfi] n. 脊髓造影术
myocardium [ˌmaiə'kɑ:diəm] n. 心肌

N

necrosis [ne'krəusis] n. 坏死;复数 necroses [ne'krəusi:z]
negative predictive value 阴性预测值
neoplasm ['ni(:)əuplæzəm] n. 新生物、肿瘤
neurosurgery ['njuərəusə:dʒəri] n. 神经外科学
nipple ['nipl] n. 乳头
nit [nit] n. 尼特(表面亮度单位)
no significant differences 无显著差异
no statistical differences were observed between…and… ……与……之间未见统计学差异
no statistically significant differences 无统计学差异
nodule ['nɔdju:l] n. 结、小结
noise [nɔiz] n. 噪声
noninvasive [ˌnɔnin'veisiv] a. 非侵袭的
nonionic contrast material 非离子型对比剂
nonspiral CT 非螺旋 CT
noticeably ad. 引人注意地、显著地
novel ['nɔvl] a. 新颖的
nuclear ['nju:kliə] a.(原子)核的
numerous ['nju:mərəs] a. 为数众多的

O

oblique [ə'bli:k] a. 斜的,倾斜的
obscuration [ɔbskjuə'reiʃən] n. 模糊
obstruction [əb'strʌkʃən] n. 梗阻
occult [ə'kʌlt] a. 隐的、难懂的
on the assumption that 假定
oncology [ɔŋ'kɔlədʒi] n. 肿瘤学
opacification [əupæsifi'keiʃən] n. 不透光
opportunity [ˌɔpə'tju:nəti] n. 机会
optic ['ɔptik] a. 眼的
option ['ɔpʃən] n. 选择
oral contrast material 口服对比剂
orbit ['ɔ:bit] n. 眶,轨道
orbitomeatal line 听眦线
organ ['ɔ:gən] n. 器官

orientation [ˌɔ:riən'teiʃn] *n.* 定向的
orthopedic [ɔ:θəu'pi:dik] *n.* 矫形外科学
Our observations confirm that... 我们的观察证实……
outcome ['autkʌm] *n.* 结果
outpatient ['autpeiʃnt] *n.* 门诊病人
output ['autput] *n.* 效率、输出量、功率
oval ['əuvl] *a.* 卵圆的、卵形的
ovarian [əu'vɛəriən] *a.* 卵巢的
overlap [ˌəuvə'læp] *v.* 重叠

P

P value　*P* 值
pacemaker ['peismeikə] *n.* 起搏器
pancreatitis [ˌpæŋkriə'taitis] *n.* 胰腺炎
panel size 平板尺寸
pant [pænt] *n.* 气喘、心跳
papillary [pə'piləri] *a.* 乳头的、乳头状的
parameter [pə'ræmitə] *n.* 参数
paranoia [ˌpærə'nɔiə] *n.* 妄想狂、偏执狂
parenchyma [pə'reŋkimə] *n.* 实质
particular [pə'tikjulə] *a.* 特别的
pathologic [ˌpæθə'lɔdʒik] *a.* 病理的
patient ['peiʃənt] *n.* 病人、患者
peak kilovoltage 峰电压
pectoralis ['pektərəlis] *a.* 胸的
pedicle ['pedikl] *n.* 蒂
pelvis ['pelvis] *n.* 骨盆; 复数 pelvises 或 pelves
pelvic floor 盆底
penetrate ['penitreit] *v.* 透入、贯穿
perceivable *a.* 可见的
perihilar ['peraihilər] *a.* 肺门周围的
peripheral [pə'rifərəl] *a.* 外周的、周围的、末梢的
perpendicular [ˌpə:pən'dikjulə] *a.* 与……垂直的(to)
persistent [pə'sistənt] *a.* 持久的
phalanx ['fælæŋks] *n.* 指骨、趾骨; 复数 phalanges [fæ'lændʒi:z]
phantom ['fæntəm] *n.* 体模
phased array coil 相控阵列线圈
photon ['fəutɔn] *n.* 光子
phototimer ['fəutəutaimə] *n.* 曝光计
physician [fi'ziʃən] *n.* 医师
physician assistant 助理医师
physiologic [fiziə'lɔdʒik] *a.* 生理的、生理学的
picture archiving and communication systems 图像存档与传输系统,简称 PACS
pillow ['piləu] *n.* 垫枕
pilot ['pailət] *a.* 先导的
pitch [pitʃ] *n.* 螺距
plague [pleig] *vt.* 烦扰、使苦恼
plaque [plɑ:k] *n.* 斑块
plateau [plæ'təu] *n.* 平高线、平顶; 复数 plateaus 或 plateaux
play an essential role 起着必不可少的作用
pleural effusion 胸腔积液
pneumonia [nju(:)'məuniə] *n.* 肺炎
pneumothorax [ˌnju:mə'θɔ:ræks] *n.* 气胸
polarized *a.* 极化的、偏振的
porcine ['pɔ:sain] *a.* 猪的
position [pə'ziʃən] *vt.* 给……定位
positive predictive value 阳性预测值
positron emission tomography 正电子发射断层显像技术,简称 PET
posteroanterior [pɔstərəuæn'tiəriə] *a.* 后前位的
prediction [pri'dikʃən] *n.* 预言、预告
pregnancy ['pregnənsi] *n.* 妊娠、怀孕
prevail [pri'veil] *vi.* 占优势,经常发生
previous ['pri:viəs] *a.* 早先的、以前的
primary ['praiməri] *a.* 原发的
prior ['praiə] *a.* 在前的(to)

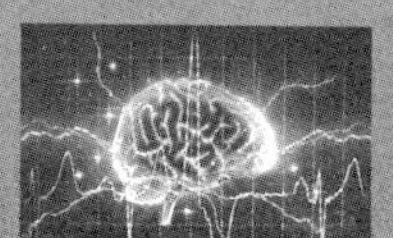

priority [prai'ɔriti] *n.* 先前
process ['prəuses, 美 'prɔses] *vt.* 加工、处理
processor ['prəusesə] *n.* 洗片机
prohibitive [prə'hibitiv] *a.* 禁止的、抑制的
projection [prə'dʒekʃən] *n.* 投射、投影
prone [prəun] *a.* 易于……的 (to)
pronounced [prə'naunst] *a.* 显著的、明显的
property ['prɔpəti] *n.* 性质、特性
proprietary [prə'praiətəri] *a.* 所有人的、专有的
prospective [prəs'pektiv] *a.* 未来的、预期的
prototype ['prəutətaip] *n.* 原型
pulmonary ['pʌlmənəri] *a.* 肺的
pulse sequence 脉冲序列
puncture ['pʌŋktʃə] *n.* 小孔
pyelocalyceal 肾盏

Q

quality control 质量控制,简称 QC

R

radiation dose 放射剂量
radiation [ˌreidi'eiʃən] *n.* 辐射、照射
radiation therapy 放射治疗
radiograph ['reidiəugrɑ:f] X 线照相
radiographic [ˌreidiəu'græfik] *a.* 放射摄影的、X 线摄影的
radiography [reidi'ɔgrəfi] *n.* X 线摄影
radiologist *n.* 放射学家
Radiology Department 放射科
radius ['reidiəs] *n.* 桡骨; 复数 radii ['reidiai]
randomize ['rændəmaiz] *vt.* 使随机化
randomly *ad.* 随机地
reader ['ri:də] *n.* 阅读器
readout layer 判读层
receiver operating characteristic curves 受试者作业特性曲线
recognition [rekəg'niʃən] *n.* 识别、认出
recommendation [ˌrekəmen'deiʃən] *n.* 建议、推荐
reconstruction [ˌri:kən'strʌkʃn] *vt.* 重建
reconstruction algorithm 重建算法
reconstruction increment 重建增量
reconstruction interval 重建间隔
redesign [ˌri:di'zain] *v.* 重新设计
reference lines 参考线
refusal [ri'fju:zl] *n.* 拒绝
region of interest 兴趣区
register ['redʒistə] *n.* 记录
Reid baseline 里德基线(连接眶下嵴至外耳道及枕区中线之线,用于测颅)
relaxation [ˌri:læk'seiʃən] *n.* 弛豫
relaxation enhancement technique 弛豫增强技术
relevant ['relivənt] *a.* 相应的
renal failure 肾衰竭
renal insufficiency 肾功能不全
repetition time 重复时间
repository [ri'pɔzətri] *n.* 仓库、资源丰富地区
residency *n.* 住院医师
resident physician 住院医师
resist [ri'zist] *v.* 阻碍
respiration ['respə'reiʃn] *n.* 呼吸
respiratory impairment 呼吸障碍
result from 由……引起
result in 导致
resultant [ri'zʌltənt] *n.* 结果
retrieve [ri'tri:v] *vt.* 重新得到、取回
retrocardiac [retrəu'kɑ:diæk] *a.* 心后的
retrograde urography 逆行性尿路造影术
retrospect *n.* 回顾、追溯
retrospective electrocardiographic gate 回顾性心电门控

revolution[ˌrevə'lu:ʃn]n. 循环、周期
rise superior to 超越
ROC curve analysis　ROC 曲线分析
root-mean-square 均方根
rotation[rəu'teiʃn]n. 旋转
routine chest radiography 常规胸部 X 线摄影
rural['ruərəl]a. 农村的
R-wave　R 波

S

sagittal['sædʒətəl]a. 矢状的
saturation[ˌsætʃə'reiʃn]n. 饱和
scan[skæn]v. 扫描
scatter radiation 散射线
schedule['ʃedju:l]vt. 计划
score[skɔ:]n. 分数
screen film mammography 屏 - 片乳腺 X 线摄影
screening['skri:niŋ]n. 筛选、审查
selective localization 选择性定位
selenium[si'li:niəm]n. 硒
semiconductor element 半导体元素
senior['si:niə]a. 年长的、资历较深的
sensitivity[sensə'tivəti]n. 灵敏(度、性)
sensor['sensə]n. 传感器、感受器
separate['sepəreit]a. v. 分离
sequence['si:kwəns]n. 连续、顺序、定序
serum creatinine level 血清肌酐水平
side by side 并排地、一起
sigmoid['sigmɔid]n. S 形；sigmoidal a.
silhouette[ˌsilu'et]n. 轮廓、侧面影像、剪影
silicon['silikən]n. 硅
simulate['simjuleit]vt. 模拟、仿真、假装
similar['similə]a. 相似的
single-detector row spiral CT 单排探测器螺旋 CT
single-segment image reconstruction 单扇区影像重建
single-shot turbo spin-echo sequence 单次激发快速自旋回波序列
skeletal['skelətl]a. 骨骼的
skin[skin]n. 皮肤
skull[skʌl]n. 头颅骨
slice thickness 层厚
slot-scanning 裂隙扫描
small bowel 小肠
sodium chloride 氯化钠
soft-copy 软拷贝
soft-copy display 软拷贝显示
soft-tissue algorithm 软组织算法
soft-tissue window 软组织窗
solely ad. 独自、完全
solid-state a. 固态的、硬的
somewhat similar to 有点类似于
sonographic['səunəu'græfik]a. 超声检查的
sonography[səu'nɔgrəfi]n. 超声检查
source[sɔ:s]n. 源、出处
spatial resolution 空间分辨率
Spearman correlation analysis　Spearman 相关分析
specificity[ˌspesi'fisəti]n. 特异性
specimen['spesimən]n. 标本、抽样
spine[spain]n. 棘、脊柱
spotlight['spɔtlait]聚光灯
stabilize['steibəlaiz]vt. 使稳定
stair-step artifcts 阶梯状伪影
static['stætik]a. 静止的,固定的
stationary grid 固定滤线栅
statistical analysis software 统计分析软件,简称 SAS
statistically significant difference 显著的统计学差异
stenosis[sti'nəusis]n. 狭 窄; 复 数 stenoses

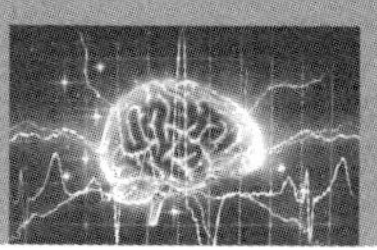

[sti'nəusi:z]

stereotaxic [ˌsteri:əu'tæksik] *a.* 立体定位的

stimulate ['stimjuleit] *vt.* 刺激

storage phosphor plate 存储荧光板

strategy ['strætədʒi] *n.* 战略、对策

streak-emitting shadows 条纹放射影

strength [streŋθ] *n.* 强度、力量、浓度

structure ['strʌktʃə] *n.* 结构

Student's *t* test for paired samples 配对 *t* 检验

subdue [səb'dju:] *vt.* 减弱、使光线柔和

subjective [sʌb'dʒektiv] *a.* 主观的

subjective assessment 主观评价

submit [səb'mit] *v.* 提交

subsequent ['sʌbsikwənt] *a.* 后来的

subspecialty [sʌb'speʃəlti] *n.* 亚专科

substantial [səb'stænʃəl] *a.* 物质的、实际的、坚固的、重要的

subtle ['sʌtl] *a.* 微妙的、细微的

subtract [səb'trækt] *v.* 减去

subtraction [səb'trækʃn] *n.* 减去

suitable ['sju:təbl] *a.* 合适的、适宜的、适当的

superimpose [ˌsu:pərim'pəuz] *vt.* 把……放在另一物的上面、附加

superior [su:'piəriə] *a.* 上等的,在上的,占优的

supplant [sə'plɑ:nt] *vt.* 取代

suppression [sə'preʃən] *n.* 抑制

supraorbitomeatal line 眶上线

surface coil 表面线圈

surgery ['sə:dʒəri] *n.* 外科、外科学

suspect [səs'pekt] *vt.* 怀疑

sweep [swi:p](swept, swept) *v.* 扫描

symmetry ['simətri] *n.* 对称

symptomatic [ˌsimptə'mætik] *a.* 有症状的

synchronization [ˌsiŋkrənai'zeiʃn] *n.* 同步、使时间一致

synchronously ['siŋkrənəsli] *ad.* 同时发生地、同步地

synthesis ['sinθisis] *n.* 合成; 复数 syntheses ['sinθisi:z]

system ['sistim 'sistəm] *n.* 系统

systole ['sistəli] *n.* 收缩期

T

T_1-weighted imaging　T_1 加权成像

table speed 床速

take a biopsy 做活检

tarsal ['tɑ:səl] *n.* 跗骨

tear [tɛə] *vt.* 撕、损伤; tore torn

technologist *n.* 技术人员(专家)

tedium ['ti:diəm] *n.* 单调、冗长乏味、沉闷

teleradiology 远程放射学

temporal resolution 时间分辨率

temporal subtraction 时间减影

temporal subtraction image 时间减影图像

temporal ['tempərəl] *a.* 瞬时的、短暂的

the dose level 剂量水平

the world wide web 万维网

theoretical [θiə'retikəl] *a.* 理论上的

therapy ['θerəpi] *n.* 治疗

thoracic [θɔ:'ræsik] *a.* 胸的、胸廓的

thoracoabdominal [θɔ:rə'kəuəbdəminl] *a.* 胸腹的

thorax ['θɔ:ræks] *n.* 胸,胸廓; 复数 thoraxes 或 thoraces ['θɔ:rəsi:z]

throughput [θru:'put] *n.* 通过量、吞吐量

tibia ['tibiə] *n.* 胫骨; 复数 tibias 或 tibiae ['tibii:]

to have no effect, without effect 无效

to the advantage of 对……有利

to the best effect 最有效地

topogram *n.* top 像

trabecula [trə'bekjulə] *n.* 小梁; 复数 trabeculae

[trə'bekjuli:]
trachea ['treikiə, trə'ki(:)ə] n. 气 管; 复 数 tracheas 或 tracheae ['treikii:, trə'ki:i:]
tracheal a. 气管的
tract [trækt] n. 道
trade-off n. 折中、权衡
transfer ['trænsfə:] (transferred, transferring) v. 传输
transmission [træns'miʃən] n. 透射、发射、传输
trap [træp] n. 陷阱
trauma ['trɔ:mə] (复 数 traumas 或 traumata) n. 损伤、外伤、创伤
tremendous [trə'mendəs] a. 可怕的、惊人的
triphase ['traifeiz] a. 三相的
tripod ['traipɔd] n. 三脚架
troubleshoot ['trʌblʃu:t] 消除缺陷、发现缺点
tube [tju:b] n. 球管
tube current 管电流
tube voltage 管电压
tumor ['tju:mə] n. 肿瘤
turbo spin echo 快速自旋回波
two-segment reconstruction 双扇区重建

U

uniformity [ˌju:ni'fɔ:məti] n. 均匀(性、度)
uptake ['ʌpteik] n. 摄入、摄取
ureter [ju'ri:tə] n. 输尿管
urinary ['juərinəri] a. 尿的、泌尿的
urography [juə'rɔgrəfi] n. 尿路造影术
urologic [juərəu'lɔdʒik] a. 泌尿科的

V

validate ['vælideit] vt. 确认、证实
vascular ['væskjulə] a. 血管的、脉管的
vast [vɑ:st] a. 巨大的
veil [veil] n. 模糊、遮蔽物
venous ['vi:nəs] a. 静脉的
ventilation [venti'leiʃən] n. 通气
versatile ['və:sətail] a. 通用的、万能的
vessel ['vesl] n. 管、脉管
vice versa ['vɑisi 'və:sə] 反之亦然
viewing conditions 观片条件
visibility of anatomic structures 解剖结构的可见度
volume render 容积再现
volunteer [vɔlən'tiə] n. 自愿者
vulnerability [vʌlnərə'biliti] n. 弱点

W

We believe that... 我们认为……
We conclude that... 我们的结论是……
We suggest that... 我们建议……
weakness n. 虚弱
whole-body imager 全身成像仪
window level 窗位
window width 窗宽
with effect 有效
withdrawal [wið'drɔ:əl] n. 收回、撤销
work flow 工作流程
workplace n. 工作场所
wrist [rist] n. 腕

X

xenon ['zenɔn] n. 氙
X-ray tube X 线管

Z

zoom [zu:m] n. 图像电子放大

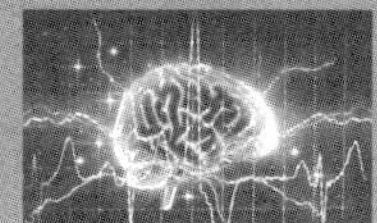

附录 B

赫尔辛基宣言
（*The Declaration of Helsinki*）

世界医学协会赫尔辛基宣言涉及人体对象医学研究的道德原则经第 18 届世界医学协会联合大会（赫尔辛基，芬兰，1964 年 6 月）采用，并由下列联合大会修改。

第 29 届世界医学协会联合大会，东京，日本，1975 年 10 月；

第 35 届世界医学协会联合大会，威尼斯，意大利，1983 年 10 月；

第 41 届世界医学协会联合大会，香港，中国，1989 年 9 月；

第 48 届世界医学协会联合大会，西萨默塞特，南非，1996 年 10 月；

第 52 届世界医学协会联合大会，爱丁堡，苏格兰，2000 年 10 月；

第 59 届世界医学协会联合大会，首尔，韩国，2008 年。

A. 前 言

1. 世界医学协会（WMA）制定《赫尔辛基宣言》，是作为关于涉及人类受试者的医学研究，包括对可确定的人体材料和数据的研究，是有关伦理原则的一项声明。《宣言》应整体阅读，其每一段落应在顾及所有其他相关段落的情况下方可运用。

2. 尽管《宣言》主要针对医生，世界医学协会鼓励涉及人类受试者的医学研究的其他参与者接受这些原则。

3. 促进和保护患者的健康，包括那些参与医学研究的患者，是医生的责任。医生的知识和良心奉献于实现这一责任。

4. 世界医学协会的《日内瓦宣言》用下列词语约束医生，“患者的健康为我最首先要考虑的”，《国际医学伦理标准》宣告，“医生在提供医护时应从患者的最佳利益出发”。

5. 医学进步是以最终必须包括涉及人类受试者的研究为基础的。应为那些在医学研究没有涉及的人口提供机会，使他们参与研究之中。

6. 在涉及人类受试者的医学研究中，个体研究受试者的福祉必须高于所有其他利益。

7. 涉及人类受试者的医学研究的基本目的，是了解疾病起因、发展和影响，并改进预防、诊断和治疗干预措施(方法、操作和治疗)。即使对当前最佳干预措施也必须不断通过研究,对其安全、效力、功效、可及性和质量给予评估。

8. 在医学实践和医学研究中,大多干预措施具有危险,会造成负担。

9. 医学研究要符合促进尊重所有人类受试者、保护他们健康和权利的伦理标准。一些研究涉及的人口尤其脆弱,需要特别保护。这包括那些自己不能给予或拒绝同意意见的人口和那些有可能被强迫或受到不正当影响的人口。

10. 医生在开展涉及人类受试者的研究时应不仅考虑本国的伦理的、法律的和规定的规范和标准,也要考虑适用的国际规范和标准。国家的伦理的、法律的和规定的要求不应减少或排除本《宣言》制定的对研究受试者的任何保护条款。

B. 所有医学研究适用的原则

11. 参与医学研究的医生有责任保护研究受试者的生命、健康、尊严、公正、自我决定的权利、隐私和个人信息的保密。

12. 涉及人类受试者的医学研究应符合普遍认可的科学原则,以对科学文献、其他适宜信息、足够实验信息和适宜动物实验信息的充分了解为基础。实验用动物的福利应给予尊重。

13. 开展有可能损害环境的试验时应适当谨慎。

14. 每个涉及人类受试者的研究项目的设计和操作,应在研究规程中有明确的描述。研究规程应包括一项关于伦理考虑的表达,应表明本《宣言》中原则是如何得到体现的。研究规程应包括有关资金来源、赞助者、组织隶属单位、其他潜在利益冲突、对研究受试者的激励措施,以及参与研究造成伤害的治疗和(或)补偿条款等。研究规程应描述研究项目结束后研究受试者可以得到有利于研究受试者的干预措施安排,或可以得到其他适宜医护或好处的安排。

15. 在研究开始前,研究规程必须提交给研究伦理委员会,供其考虑、评论、指导和同意。该委员会必须独立于研究人员、赞助者和任何不正当影响之外。该委员会必须考虑到研究项目开展国家或各国的法律和规定,以及适用的国际规范和标准,但是这些决不允许减少或消除本《宣言》为研究受试者制定的保护条款。该委员会必须有权监督研究的开展。研究人员必须向该委员会提供监督的信息,特别是关于严重负面事件的信息。未经该委员会的考虑和批准,不可对研究规程进行修改。

16. 涉及人类受试者的医学研究必须仅限受过适当科学培训和具备资格的人员来开展。对患者或健康志愿者的研究要求由一名胜任的、符合资格的医生负责监督管理。保护研究受试者的责任必须总是属于这名医生或其他卫生保健专业人员,决不能属于研究受试者,即使他们同意。

17. 涉及弱势或脆弱人口或社区的医学研究,只有在研究是为这类人口或社区的健康需要、是他们的优先项目时,以及有理由相信这类人口或社区可能从该研究结果中获得益处

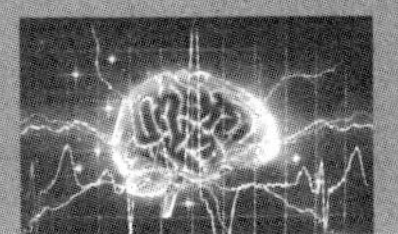

时，方可开展。

18. 每个涉及人类受试者的医学研究项目在开展前，必须对其可预见的对参与研究的个人和社区造成的危险和负担，做出谨慎的评估，与可预见的对他们或其他受研究影响的个人或社区的好处进行对比。

19. 每次临床试验在征用第一位研究对象前，必须在公众可及的数据库登记。

20. 医生不可参与涉及人类受试者的医学研究，除非他们有信心相信对可能造成的危险已做过足够的评估，并可以得到令人满意的管理。当医生发现一项研究的危险会大于潜在益处，或当已得到研究的正面和有益结论性证明后，必须立即停止该项研究。

21. 涉及人类受试者的医学研究仅可以在目的重要性高于对研究受试者的内在危险和负担的情况下才能开展。

22. 合格的个人作为受试者参与医学研究必须是自愿的。尽管可能与家人或社区负责人商议是适当的，但是即使是合格的个人也不可被招募用于研究项目，除非他（她）自由表达同意。

23. 必须采取一切措施保护研究受试者的隐私和为个人信息保密，并使研究最低限度对他们的身体、精神和社会地位造成影响。

24. 涉及合格的人类受试者的医学研究，每位潜在受试者必须得到足够的有关研究目的、方法、资金来源、任何可能的利益冲突、研究人员的组织隶属、研究期望的好处和潜在危险、研究可能造成的不适以及任何其他相关方面的信息。潜在研究受试者必须被告知其可以拒绝参加研究的权利，或在研究过程中任何时间推翻同意意见而退出并不会被报复的权利。特别应注意为潜在研究受试者个人提供他们所需的具体信息，以及使其了解提供信息的方法。在确保潜在研究受试者理解了信息后，医生或其他一位适当的有资格的人必须寻求潜在研究受试者自由表达的知情同意，最好为书面形式。如果同意的意见不能用书面表达，非书面同意意见应被正式记录并有证人目击。

25. 对于使用可确认的人体材料或数据的医学研究，医生通常必须寻求对收集、分析、存放和（或）再使用的同意意见。可能会有不可能，或不现实，为研究得到同意意见的情况，或会有为研究得到同意意见会为研究的有效性造成威胁的情况。在这些情况下，只有在一个研究伦理委员会的考虑和同意后，研究方可进行。

26. 在寻求参与研究项目的知情同意时，如果潜在受试者与医生有依赖关系，或可能会被迫表示同意，医生应特别谨慎。在这些情况下，应该由一位适当的有资格且完全独立于这种关系之外的人来寻求知情同意。

27. 如果潜在研究受试者不具备能力，医生必须寻求法律上被授权的代表的知情同意。这些不具备能力的潜在研究受试者决不能被介入到对他们没有益处可能的研究中，除非研究项目的目的是促进该潜在受试者所代表的人口的健康，而且研究又缺少具备能力人员的参与，而且研究只会使潜在受试者承受最低限度的危险和最小的负担。

28. 当一位被认为不具备能力的潜在研究受试者实际有能力做出同意参与研究的决定时，医生应除寻求法律上被授权代表的同意外，还必须寻求研究受试者的同意。潜在受试者做出不同意的意见应予尊重。

29. 研究涉及那些身体上或精神上不具备做出同意意见的能力时，比如无意识的患者，应只有在阻碍给予知情同意意见的身体或精神状况正是被研究人口的一个必要特点时才可以开展。在这种情况下，医生应寻求法律上被授权代表的知情同意。如果缺少此类代表，而且研究不能延误，如果参与研究的受试者处在无法给予知情同意的状况下这些具体理由已在研究规程中陈述，该研究已得到研究伦理委员会的批准则研究项目没有知情同意可以开展。同意继续参与研究的意见应尽早从研究受试者或法律上被授权代表那里获得。

30. 作者、编辑和出版者对于出版研究成果都有伦理义务。作者有责任公开他们涉及人类受试者的研究成果并对其报告的完整和准确性负责。他们应遵守已被接受的伦理报告指导方针。负面和非结论性结果应同正面的结果一样发表，或通过其他途径使公众可以得到。资金来源、机构隶属及利益冲突等应在出版物上宣布。不遵守本《宣言》原则的研究报告不应被接受发表。

C. 有关与医护相结合的医学研究的其他原则

31. 只有当研究潜在的预防、诊断或治疗的价值足以说明研究的必要性，而且医生有充分理由相信参与研究不会对作为研究受试者的患者的健康带来负面影响时，医生才可以把医学研究与医护相结合。

32. 一种新干预措施的益处、危险、负担、有效性等，必须与当前被证明最佳干预措施进行对照试验，除非在下列情况下：

——在当前没有被证明有效的干预措施情况下，研究中使用安慰剂，或无治疗处理，是可以接受的。

——在有紧迫和科学得当方法方面的理由上相信，使用安慰剂是必要的，以便确定一种干预措施的功效或安全性，而且使用安慰剂或无治疗处理的患者不会受到任何严重或不可逆转伤害危险的情况下。对这种选择必须极其谨慎以避免滥用。

33. 在研究项目结束时，参与研究的患者有权得知研究的结果并分享由此产生的任何益处，比如有权接受研究中确认有效的干预措施或其他适当的医护或益处。

34. 医生必须向患者全面通报医护的哪些方面与研究项目有关。患者拒绝参与研究或决定退出研究，绝不能妨碍患者 - 医生关系。

35. 在治疗一名患者时，如果没有被证明有效的干预措施，或有被证明无效的干预措施，医生在寻求专家意见后，并得到患者或法律上被授权代表的知情同意后，如果根据医生的判断，这个未被证明有效的干预措施有希望挽救生命、重建健康或减少痛苦。则可以使用此干预措施，在可能情况下，这个干预措施应作为研究的目的，设计成可评估它的安全性和有效性。在所有情况下，新信息应被记录，并在适当时公布于众。

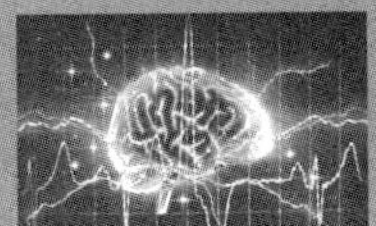

A. INTRODUCTION

1. The World Medical Association (WMA) has developed *the Declaration of Helsinki* as a statement of ethical principles for medical research involving human subjects, including research on identifiable human material and data. The Declaration is intended to be read as a whole and each of its constituent paragraphs should not be applied without consideration of all otherrelevant paragraphs.

2. Although the Declaration is addressed primarily to physicians, the WMA encourages other participants in medical research involving human subjects to adopt these principles.

3. It is the duty of the physician to promote and safeguard the health of patients, including those who are involved in medical research. The physician's knowledge and conscience are dedicated to the fulfilment of this duty.

4. The Declaration of Geneva of the WMA binds the physician with the words, "The health of my patient will be my first consideration" , and the International Code of Medical Ethics declares that, "A physician shall act in the patient's best interest when providing medical care" .

5. Medical progress is based on research that ultimately must include studies involving human subjects. Populations that are underrepresented in medical research should be provided appropriate access to participation in research.

6. In medical research involving human subjects, the well-being of the individual research subject must take precedence over all other interests.

7. The primary purpose of medical research involving human subjects is to understand the causes, development and effects of diseases and improve preventive, diagnostic and therapeutic interventions (methods, procedures and treatments). Even the best current interventions must be evaluated continually through research for their safety, effectiveness, efficiency, accessibility and quality.

8. In medical practice and in medical research, most interventions involve risks and burdens.

9. Medical research is subject to ethical standards that promote respect for all human subjects and protect their health and rights. Some research populations are particularly vulnerable and need special protection. These include those who cannot give or refuse consent for themselves and those who may be vulnerable to coercion or undue influence.

10. Physicians should consider the ethical, legal and regulatory norms and standards for research involving human subjects in their own countries as well as applicable international norms and standards. No national or international ethical, legal or regulatory requirement should reduce or eliminate any of the protections for research subjects set forth in this Declaration.

B. BASIC PRINCIPLES FOR ALL MEDICAL RESEARCH

11. It is the duty of physicians who participate in medical research to protect the life, health, dignity, integrity, right to self-determination, privacy, and confidentiality of personal information of research subjects.

12. Medical research involving human subjects must conform to generally accepted scientific principles, be based on a thorough knowledge of the scientific literature, other relevant sources of information, and adequate laboratory and, as appropriate, animal experimentation. The welfare of animals used for research must be respected.

13. Appropriate caution must be exercised in the conduct of medical research that may harm the environment.

14. The design and performance of each research study involving human subjects must be clearly described in a research protocol. The protocol should contain a statement of the ethical considerations involved and should indicate how the principles in this Declaration have been addressed. The protocol should include information regarding funding, sponsors, institutional affiliations, other potential conflicts of interest, incentives for subjects and provisions for treating and/or compensating subjects who are harmed as a consequence of participation in the research study. The protocol should describe arrangements for post-study access by study subjects to interventions identified as beneficial in the study or access to other appropriate care or benefits.

15. The research protocol must be submitted for consideration, comment, guidance and approval to a research ethics committee before the study begins. This committee must be independent of the researcher, the sponsor and any other undue influence. It must take into consideration the laws and regulations of the country or countries in which the research is to be performed as well as applicable international norms and standards but these must not be allowed to reduce or eliminate any of the protections for research subjects set forth in this Declaration. The committee must have the right to monitor ongoing studies. The researcher must provide monitoring information to the committee, especially information about any serious adverse events. No change to the protocol may be made without consideration and approval by the committee.

16. Medical research involving human subjects must be conducted only by individuals with the appropriate scientific training and qualifications. Research on patients or healthy volunteers requires the supervision of a competent and appropriately qualified physician or other health care professional. The responsibility for the protection of research subjects must always rest with the physician or other health care professional and never the research subjects, even though they have given consent.

17. Medical research involving a disadvantaged or vulnerable population or community is only justified if the research is responsive to the health needs and priorities of this population or

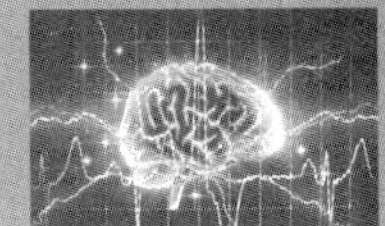

community and if there is a reasonable likelihood that this population or community stands to benefit from the results of the research.

18. Every medical research study involving human subjects must be preceded by careful assessment of predictable risks and burdens to the individuals and communities involved in the research in comparison with foreseeable benefits to them and to other individuals or communities affected by the condition under investigation.

19. Every clinical trial must be registered in a publicly accessible database before recruitment of the first subject.

20. Physicians may not participate in a research study involving human subjects unless they are confident that the risks involved have been adequately assessed and can be satisfactorily managed. Physicians must immediately stop a study when the risks are found to outweigh the potential benefits or when there is conclusive proof of positive and beneficial results.

21. Medical research involving human subjects may only be conducted if the importance of the objective outweighs the inherent risks and burdens to the research subjects.

22. Participation by competent individuals as subjects in medical research must be voluntary. Although it may be appropriate to consult family members or community leaders, no competent individual may be enrolled in a research study unless he or she freely agrees.

23. Every precaution must be taken to protect the privacy of research subjects and the confidentiality of their personal information and to minimize the impact of the study on their physical, mental and social integrity.

24. In medical research involving competent human subjects, each potential subject must be adequately informed of the aims, methods, sources of funding, any possible conflicts of interest, institutional affiliations of the researcher, the anticipated benefits and potential risks of the study and the discomfort it may entail, and any other relevant aspects of the study. The potential subject must be informed of the right to refuse to participate in the study or to withdraw consent to participate at any time without reprisal. Special attention should be given to the specific information needs of individual potential subjects as well as to the methods used to deliver the information. After ensuring that the potential subject has understood the information, the physician or another appropriately qualified individual must then seek the potential subject's freely-given informed consent, preferably in writing. If the consent cannot be expressed in writing, the non-written consent must be formally documented and witnessed.

25. For medical research using identifiable human material or data, physicians must normally seek consent for the collection, analysis, storage and/or reuse. There may be situations where consent would be impossible or impractical to obtain for such research or would pose a threat to the validity of the research. In such situations the research may be done only after consideration and approval of a research ethics committee.

26. When seeking informed consent for participation in a research study the physician should be particularly cautious if the potential subject is in a dependent relationship with the physician or may consent under duress. In such situations the informed consent should be sought by an appropriately qualified individual who is completely independent of this relationship.

27. For a potential research subject who is incompetent, the physician must seek informed consent from the legally authorized representative. These individuals must not be included in a research study that has no likelihood of benefit for them unless it is intended to promote the health of the population represented by the potential subject, the research cannot instead be performed with competent persons, and the research entails only minimal risk and minimal burden.

28. When a potential research subject who is deemed incompetent is able to give assent to decisions about participation in research, the physician must seek that assent in addition to the consent of the legally authorized representative. The potential subject's dissent should be respected.

29. Research involving subjects who are physically or mentally incapable of giving consent, for example, unconscious patients, may be done only if the physical or mental condition that prevents giving informed consent is a necessary characteristic of the research population. In such circumstances the physician should seek informed consent from the legally authorized representative. If no such representative is available and if the research cannot be delayed, the study may proceed without informed consent provided that the specific reasons for involving subjects with a condition that renders them unable to give informed consent have been stated in the research protocol and the study has been approved by a research ethics committee. Consent to remain in the research should be obtained as soon as possible from the subject or a legally authorized representative.

30. Authors, editors and publishers all have ethical obligations with regard to the publication of the results of research. Authors have a duty to make publicly available the results of their research on human subjects and are accountable for the completeness and accuracy of their reports. They should adhere to accepted guidelines for ethical reporting. Negative and inconclusive as well as positive results should be published or otherwise made publicly available. Sources of funding, institutional affiliations and conflicts of interest should be declared in the publication. Reports of research not in accordance with the principles of this Declaration should not be accepted for publication.

C. ADDITIONAL PRINCIPLES FOR MEDICAL RESEARCH COMBINED WITH MEDICAL CARE

31. The physician may combine medical research with medical care only to the extent that the research is justified by its potential preventive, diagnostic or therapeutic value and if the

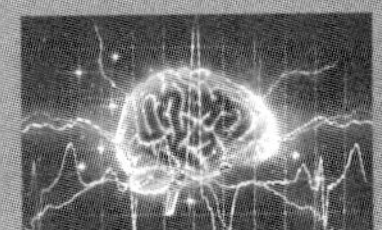

physician has good reason to believe that participation in the research study will not adversely affect the health of the patients who serve as research subjects.

32. The benefits, risks, burdens and effectiveness of a new intervention must be tested against those of the best current proven intervention, except in the following circumstances: The use of placebo, or no treatment, is acceptable in studies where no current proven intervention exists; or Where for compelling and scientifically sound methodological reasons the use of placebo is necessary to determine the efficacy or safety of an intervention and the patients who receive placebo or no treatment will not be subject to any risk of serious or irreversible harm. Extreme care must be taken to avoid abuse of this option.

33. At the conclusion of the study, patients entered into the study are entitled to be informed about the outcome of the study and to share any benefits that result from it, for example, access to interventions identified as beneficial in the study or to other appropriate care or benefits.

34. The physician must fully inform the patient which aspects of the care are related to the research. The refusal of a patient to participate in a study or the patient's decision to withdraw from the study must never interfere with the patient-physician relationship.

35. In the treatment of a patient, where proven interventions do not exist or have been ineffective, the physician, after seeking expert advice, with informed consent from the patient or a legally authorized representative, may use an unproven intervention if in the physician's judgement it offers hope of saving life, re-establishing health or alleviating suffering. Where possible, this intervention should be made the object of research, designed to evaluate its safety and efficacy. In all cases, new information should be recorded and, where appropriate, made publicly available.